HEPATITIS C

A Do-It-Yourself Guide for Health

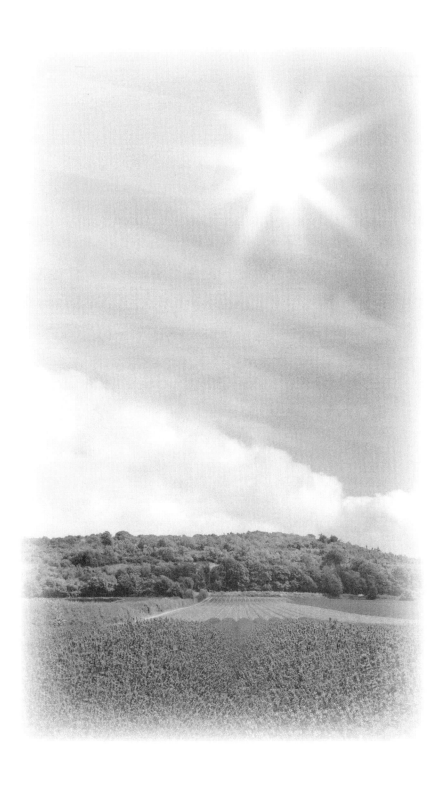

HEPATITIS C

A Do-It-Yourself Guide for Health

LLOYD WRIGHT

Lloyd Wright Publishing
Malibu, California

HEPATITIS C
A Do-It-Yourself Guide for Health
By Lloyd Wright

ISBN: 978-0-9676404-5-7

Published by Lloyd Wright Publishing
11077 Pacific View Road, Malibu, California 90265
Toll-Free: 877-676-1615   Fax: 310-457-9449
www.AlternativeMedicineSolution.com
Contact the author at Lloyd@HepatitisCFree.com

Editor: David Drum
Book cover and interior design:
Peri Poloni-Gabriel, Knockout Design, www.knockoutbooks.com

Printed in the United States of America

11 12 13 14 15 16   7 6 5 4 3 2 1

DISCLAIMER:
Please Read Carefully

The reader or purchaser of this book hereby acknowledges receiving notification by means of this disclaimer that all opinions, observations, and recommendations expressed herein are solely those of the author and should be construed neither as statements of scientific, medical, or historical fact, nor as medical advice. Anyone with questions regarding the success of the products and regimens described herein is invited to contact the author by mail, phone, fax, or e-mail (please see bottom of previous page). Anyone who purchases this book, or any of the supplements described herein, acknowledges that they are doing so on the basis of their own investigation, and not solely on the information provided herein or in any product literature related to these supplements.

Hepatitis C is a potentially fatal disease, and persons diagnosed with it should discuss the information in this book thoroughly with their physician or other healthcare professional before utilizing the alternative care methods discussed herein.

TABLE OF CONTENTS

Chapter 1:

A TIME OF ENLIGHTENMENT

One day in 1979 I sat firmly at the controls of my bulldozer, sculpting the crest of a steep slope at my home in the Santa Monica Mountains, not far from the Pacific Ocean in Southern California. Suddenly, the hydraulic reverse system failed. Despite my frantic attempts to halt the mechanical beast, it lurched backward, flipped over on me, and tumbled down a 1,000-foot cliff after crushing me beneath its 16,000 pounds of steel.

I was in a remote area. Blood gushed from my leg. There were no houses, no buildings of any kind, for miles. Miraculously, a neighbor riding his horse saw me from a great distance and used his citizen's band radio to call for help. He contacted the local fire tower, and a medevac helicopter whisked me away to a hospital, where a doctor told me that because of my massive crush injury I was going to die from kidney failure. During the next 30 days, I underwent nine major surgeries to reattach my leg. I also received four blood transfusions, at least one of which—unbeknownst to me or my doctors—was tainted with the deadly hepatitis C virus (HCV).

In 1991, I was diagnosed with testicular cancer, the Lance Armstrong disease. I was tested for hepatitis C. The results were negative. I had the disease but the test used at that time was inaccurate. A more accurate test was introduced just months later, but my doctor did not ask to retest me. He didn't even mention that a new test was available. But, as my liver count soared, he accused me of being a hard-drinking drug-user, an accusation he had made previously when I complained of extreme fatigue and other problems.

I was a homebuilder, and I loved my work. But instead of working 12-hour days, now I found I could barely work at all. My fingernails became brittle and broke easily. My hair fell out. I had dizzy spells during the day and night sweats that soaked my bed. My doctor told me I probably needed a good rest. Another doctor said I had too much iron in my blood and sent me to a blood bank once a week to have therapeutic phlebotomies (blood removed). Fortunately, someone at the blood bank inadvertently put my blood with the donated blood, and it was tested. Two months later, I received a letter telling me I could no longer donate blood because I had hepatitis C.

I called the blood bank and spoke to a technician, who told me that I could expect to die a slow, excruciating death from hepatitis C, which would manifest itself as internal bleeding, flu-like symptoms, and hepatocellular carcinoma—primary liver cancer. He said there was no cure.

But a medical doctor told me there was a drug that supposedly could cure hepatitis C. The doctor told me that interferon alfa-2B recombinant was approved by the Food and Drug Administration (FDA) for the treatment of hepatitis C. In fact, it was the *only* FDA-approved medication for hepatitis C.

Interferon was the big drug breakthrough back then. Interferon allegedly had an 81% cure rate for hepatitis C without any serious side effects, according to the package insert. I was told to inject three million units of this drug into my body every other day.

In just one week, I turned into a monstrous beast. I was constantly enraged, hostile and violently tormented. My brain felt like it was exploding; anguish became my existence. Often, I would find myself curled up in a fetal position. Some parts of my body were on fire, while others were ice cold. I was bedridden for days. When I reported these side effects, my doctor told me to cut the dosage in half. But after 10 more weeks of taking half doses of interferon, I was sicker than ever.

I saw many medical doctors—highly recommended experts in the field who practiced at some of the biggest and most prestigious hospitals in Los Angeles. I was shocked to discover that they were indifferent to my reaction to interferon. Instead, they were using fear to frighten patients into taking this medication. We patients were told that we would suffer all sorts of horrendous and diabolical afflictions and die from liver cancer if we did not take this drug.

I escaped this fate by avoiding toxic materials and consuming whenever possible organic herbs, foods and supplements discussed in this book.

In desperation, I bought a computer and spent hours looking up information on the internet about hepatitis C. To my surprise, I discovered that much work with other treatments was being done in foreign countries, with positive results. But in the U.S. interferon remained the only treatment.

After much research, and with the help of a few dedicated experts on alternative health, I was able to conquer hepatitis C through a diet of natural foods, supplements, Natcell Thymus and a solid positive attitude. Today, I have regained my health and feel completely normal.

My triumph over hepatitis C was due to a specific program of foods and supplements. In this book, you will learn about these foods and supplements and how they are grown and processed, which in turn determine how much benefit they yield to your body. Long ago, Hippocrates (460-377 B.C.), the father of medical science, insisted that nature was the healer. Hippocrates treated his patients with proper diet, herbs, fresh air, a change of climate, and attention to habits and living conditions.

Understand that it is not actually the herb or supplement alone that heals you; it is your own strengthened immune system that monitors and protects your body. It was a combination of eating the right foods, taking key supplements, and avoiding certain drugs, all vaccines (especially hepatitis A and B and the flu shots), and many other common items often recommended to victims of hepatitis C that enabled me to beat hepatitis C. You must fuel your immune system with what it needs to do the job.

Please keep in mind that because no two people react exactly the same way to any herb or supplement, you need to become intuitive. Develop your sensitivity to what you are ingesting. Make adjustments as necessary.

You can, and must, take responsibility for your health. If you are suffering from hepatitis C, you can reclaim your health, get out of bed, get off the couch, forget about disability, and go back to work.

I published my first book back in 1999. All I wanted to do was to let people know there was a better way to deal with hepatitis C than the medical community wants you to know. I had to learn how to sell books, a whole new thing for me. But after developing a simple website to offer *Triumph Over Hepatitis C*, the next thing I knew, it was a best-seller and many people wanted to use my program.

Twelve years later, my original treatment is still working for people who are looking for the restoration of their health. Over the years, I learned many new things that would cover many volumes. I am including my best current information here.

I hope with all my heart that this approach will do the same for you; that you, too, can Triumph Over Hepatitis C.

LLOYD WRIGHT
June, 2011

MY HEALING JOURNEY

During my own recovery from hepatitis C, I took the following supplements, vitamins and herbs as part of a treatment strategy outlined in this book.

- Two 200 mg. organic *milk thistle* capsules three times a day. I also drank one quart of milk thistle tea several days a week.

- One vial of **Natcell Thymus** on an empty stomach every other day for 18 months. I also took two 500 mg. of thymus organic capsules three times a day.

- One 300 mg. *adrenal* organic capsule two times a day. I suggest taking **Natcell Adrenal**, one vial a week (optional).

- Two 500 mg. *Liver* organic capsules two times a day. I suggest taking **Natcell Liver**, two vials a week (optional).

- Two cups of *reishi* mushroom tea a day. You may also take *reishi* capsules; one 500 mg. three times a day.

- Two 100 mg. *alpha lipoic acid* capsules two times a day. Today, I suggest taking one 300 mg. *alpha lipoic acid* capsule two times a day.

- One 500 mg. *licorice root* capsule two times a day, five days a week. I also drank two cups of *licorice tea* a few days a week.

- One 500 mg. organic *dandelion root* capsule three times a day. I also drank one quart of *dandelion root tea* every evening.

- Two 500 mg. *cat's claw* capsules two times a day. I also drank two cups of *cat's claw tea* a few days a week.

- Four ounces of properly prepared *aloe vera* two to four times a day, usually more.

- 7000 mg. of *vitamin C* two times a day for three months. I suggest taking coral calcium with vitamin C as it helps promote an alkaline pH.

- One 200 mg. *selenium* capsule two times a day.

- One gram of *alfalfa* two times a day.

- One 5mg. tablet of **NADH** each morning on an empty stomach.

- Two capsules of *Eurocel*.

- One to two *Lipotrope* capsules three times a day.

- Organic *Barley grass* or *Pure Synergy* at least once a day.

Chapter 2:

HEPATITIS AND INTERFERON

Hepatitis is a medical term meaning inflammation of the liver. The liver is the largest organ in the human body, and capable of regenerating itself. Viral hepatitis is a fairly common set of systemic diseases that is marked by liver cell destruction, necrosis, and autolysis, all of which lead to anorexia, jaundice, and hepatomegaly or enlargement of the liver. Worldwide, it has been estimated that more than 500 million people have some form of hepatitis.

At this time, five types of viral hepatitis have been identified. Of the five viral diseases, hepatitis B and hepatitis C are most dangerous because people with these have a high risk of developing primary liver cancer or *hepatocellular carcinoma.*

ABOUT HEPATITIS

Hepatitis Type C, an undetermined type, the subject of this book, is the fastest rising form of hepatitis among Americans and it is one of the most serious. There are an estimated 170-200 million people worldwide with hepatitis C. According to the U.S. Centers for Disease Control (CDC), more than 3.2 million American men and women are chronically infected with the hepatitis C virus. Some 17,000 new hepatitis C infections are occurring every year in the United States, the CDC estimates.

The hepatitis C virus is spread blood-to-blood and most commonly acquired through blood transfusion from asymptomatic donors, although it may also be spread by the use of contaminated intravenous and tattoo needles, blood products, and non-sterile dental instruments. Developed countries now routinely screen donated blood to detect the hepatitis C virus. Hepatitis C is not a sexually-transmitted disease!

An estimated 15 percent of people clear the hepatitis C virus and never experience symptoms (spontaneous remission). For most, the hepatitis C virus becomes chronic and can lie dormant for some time. However, when liver cells begin to die (called necrosis), this leads first to scarring or fibrosis of the liver and then to a more serious advanced scarring called cirrhosis. Hepatitis C is the most common reason for liver transplants in the United States and it is associated with an alarming rise in primary liver cancer.

What makes hepatitis C so deadly is that this virus is able to hide *inside* liver cells. When the immune system attacks the hepatitis C virus, trying to do its job of protecting the body, liver cells become the unintended victims and begin to die off. Cirrhosis and cell death follow and this can present many terminal circumstances such as ascites and varices to name a few.

Hepatitis **Type B,** is serum or long-incubation hepatitis. Also increasing among HIV-positive individuals, hepatitis B accounts for up to 10% of post-transfusion viral hepatitis cases in the United States. In addition to blood transfusions, it is also transmitted in human excretions including feces, and from viruses spread by infected food preparers.

Hepatitis **Type A** is infection or short-incubation hepatitis. It is contracted from ingestion of tainted food. People with hepatitis C who also contract hepatitis A have a 40% fatality rate within 48 hours and survivors remain very ill for up to six months. Your doctor may recommend you take a vaccine against hepatitis A and hepatitis B. However, do NOT take this vaccine until you read about the effects of these vaccines in Chapter 4.

Hepatitis **Type D** is found most frequently as a complication of acute or chronic hepatitis B. The type D virus requires the hepatitis B organism's double-shelled surface antigen to replicate.

Hepatitis **Type E** was formerly grouped with type C under the name type non-A, non-B hepatitis. Hepatitis type E primarily occurs among people recently returned from an endemic area such as India, Africa, Asia, or Central America.

The progress of hepatitis may be tracked through several tests listed in the back of this book that assess the state of your liver, such as the ALT and AST liver function tests.

If you have hepatitis C, your medical doctor may recommend interferon treatment. Before you proceed, read this entire book.

ABOUT INTERFERON

Interferon is a type of protein formed in the body when cells are exposed to viruses. It is not specific to any particular type of virus. Interferon is an extremely powerful substance. Only ten molecules are said to induce resistance of a cell to viruses. However, the use of pharmaceutical interferon, usually with one or more antiviral drugs for periods of 24 or 48 weeks, and sometimes longer, is nothing less than a hauntingly savage journey.

The reactions I described in the Introduction have been experienced by countless users of interferon. Not everyone has these reactions, but every day I receive e-mails documenting the horrid, terrible effects of interferon, which are not limited to rage, fatigue and other intolerable symptoms.

Some of the many known possible side effects of interferon treatment include fever, chills, nausea, vomiting, loss of appetite, chest pain, congestive heart failure, stroke, lung disorders, decrease in kidney function, liver pain, changes of vision including a possibility of blindness in one or both eyes, cerebral atrophy, facial palsy, decreased cognitive abilities, autoimmune disorders, psoriasis, blood disorders, skin reactions, psychiatric effects including depression, insomnia, hallucinations, mania, suicidal thoughts, psychosis, and contemplation of suicide and homicide. Sober alcoholics and drug users have been known to suffer a relapse and overdose on alcohol or drugs. Women may suffer menstrual disorders, spontaneous abortions, birth defects, or become sterile. Some side effects may not reverse over time, and may cause death.

The use of pharmacological interferon is associated with a greater risk of type 2 diabetes and other blood sugar disorders, kidney failure, and various cancers, notably those affecting the pancreas, thyroid, liver and cervix. This doesn't mean that interferon *causes* any of these life-threatening diseases. Rather, it appears that pharmaceutical interferon interferes with the body's immune system, disabling our natural defenses.

Consider how interferon works. It lowers your white blood cell and platelet counts. This allows bacteria, infection, and viruses to enter the body and begin destroying it. Put simply, interferon puts the immune system to sleep.

After I published the first edition of my book, *Triumph Over Hepatitis C*, I began documenting a plethora of cases where hepatitis C carriers also had blood sugar disorders. I realized most of these people had also used interferon. Also, after interviewing many doctors, I ascertained that it is not unusual for hepatitis C patients to die from pancreatic cancer.

Many retired medical doctors, who now promote alternative treatments, have told me that, prior to the identification of the hepatitis C virus in 1989, there were many deaths from liver cancer in people who had a diagnosis of Non-A/Non-B hepatitis. Yet the connection between interferon treatment and liver cancer was never made. The incidence of liver cancer in victims of hepatitis C, which was around 10% and declining, has lately risen to 40%. This frightening increase coincides with the increased use of interferon.

In conclusion, I implore you not to use interferon. If you suffer from hepatitis C, use instead the natural solutions described in this book. If despite all this you decide to use interferon, please consider undertaking a program to boost your immune system.

Before submitting to the fear brought onto you by your doctor to use interferon, go to *www.interferon.ws* and read.

Just say NO to interferon!

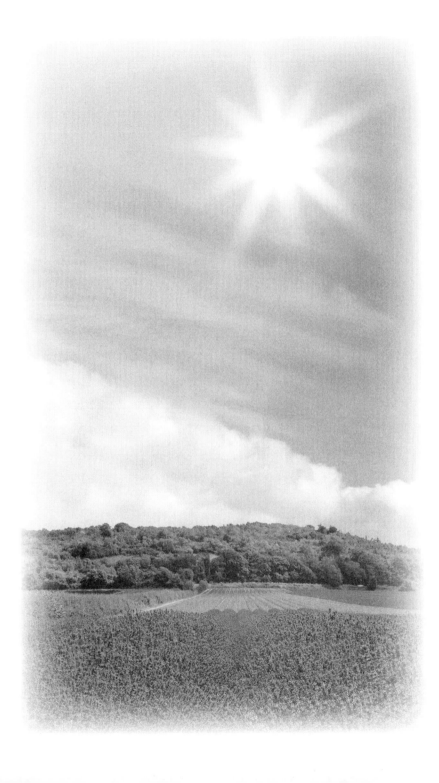

Chapter 3:

A PROGRAM FOR LIVING

M y five-part program for living involves several elements — frozen peptides and stem cells, selected supplements, vitamins, herbs, good food choices, and a generally healthy lifestyle all outlined in this chapter.

FROZEN PEPTIDES AND STEM CELLS

The most powerful group of supplements I used, Natcell Liquid Molecular Extracts, are tissue specific growth and cell signaling factor concentrates, peptides and stem cells.

These supplements are produced by Atrium Innovations, based in Quebec, Canada. Atrium has developed a patented biotechnology process to isolate and concentrate molecules in their natural, most beneficial cellular state called Natcell. This hi-tech process allows them to select desired molecules according to their size and weight and then to concentrate, bottle and flash freeze them under aseptic conditions.

Throughout this elaborate manufacturing process, the proteins are never exposed to anything but pure water. Natcell extracts are created with no heat or chemicals involved. The end-product is a natural, concentrated fresh molecular compound of the highest possible bioavailability.

NATCELL THYMUS: FOUNTAIN OF YOUTH

The thymus is a small gland located in the upper chest which has an important role in helping newborns develop immune response. It also shrinks as we age. According to immunologist Keith Kelly, the shrinkage of the thymus gland is "one of the cardinal bio-markers of aging." Over the past 40 years, science has discovered that the thymus gland is the key regulator of immunity.

Thymus gland hormones can prevent bone marrow injury and the reduction in white and red blood cell production commonly resulting from X-ray exposure, chemotherapy, and the results of a compromised liver. They can also reduce autoimmune reactions such as rheumatoid arthritis.

A large body of published clinical research on humans supports the use of gland extracts, taken orally, for a broad range of conditions including hepatitis, cancer, rheumatoid arthritis, various allergies and asthma conditions, and recurrent respiratory infections. Gland extracts have proven to be extremely non-toxic and free of side effects, with few contraindications for use.

People with advanced liver pathology will improve by using thymus extract. To reverse the progression of the hepatitis C virus, patients must incorporate the most aggressive treatment available. **Natcell frozen thymus extract feeds the human immune system what it needs to kill the hepatitis C virus. Labwork from people with HIV shows that Natcell Thymus can increase T cell activity 1000 times.**

I attribute most of the success of my own treatment for hepatitis C to the several thousand dollars I invested in this product over the course of eighteen months. My regimen consisted of taking one frozen vial every other day. *I thawed it in my hand, and poured one half of it under my tongue, held it for five minutes. Then, I repeated the process.* I also took two 500 mg. thymus organic capsules three times a day.

If I could afford the cost, I would take Natcell frozen thymus extract for the rest of my life.

NATCELL LIVER EXTRACTS: PEPTIDE GROWTH FACTORS

Natcell Liver Extract contains peptide growth factors that can limit and reverse fibrosis and cirrhosis, and are an important factor in the only treatment for ascites.

According to Stewart Lanson, M.D., of Scottsdale, Arizona, and Howard Benedikt, D.C., of New York City, both of whom practice clinical medicine and nutritional science, peptide growth factors are involved in the repair of both soft and hard body tissues, immunosuppression, enhancement of immune cellular function, improvement of bone marrow function in numerous disease states, treatment of many proliferative diseases, including the remission of cancer, the marked lowering of serum cholesterol [1], and for the elimination of all hepatitis viral diseases, but most especially for hepatitis B and C. [2]

The liver regulates many vital functions in the body by means of growth factors. Inasmuch as the liver's natural function is a part of all aspects of physical repair in the body, the peptide growth factors of the liver cells must be critical determinants of every aspect of tissue trauma or illness response. **As such, liver cell peptide growth factors have important and**

necessary therapeutic applications in the treatment of hepatitis C.

Peptide growth factors provide an essential means for a cell to communicate with its immediate environment. They act by binding to functional receptors that transduct their signals. Peptide growth factors ensure that there is a proper local homeostatic balance between the numerous cells that comprise a tissue or organ. Since a cell must adjust to changes in its environment, the cell needs mechanisms to provide this adaptation. Tissue cells, either singularly or collectively, use sets of peptide growth factors as signaling molecules to communicate with each other and to alter their own behavior to respond appropriately to their biological context.

In our interview about his use of frozen, liquid porcine liver peptide growth factors, Dr. Howard Benedikt, a nutrition-oriented chiropractor, discussed with me the potential healing benefits of these frozen liver peptides. In summary, Dr. Benedikt offered the following information about the liver's numerous growth factors:

> ✍ Growth factors have vascular functions, in that they cause the liver to store blood, regulate blood clotting, cleanse blood, discharge waste products into the bile

and aid the immune system by filtering the blood to remove bacteria and adding certain immune factors.

⚜ They have secretory functions, in that they aid digestion by synthesizing and secreting bile and keeping hormones in balance.

⚜ They have metabolic functions, in that they help to manufacture new proteins; produce quick energy; regulate fat storage; control the production and excretion of cholesterol; store certain vitamins, minerals, and sugars; metabolize alcohol, carbohydrates, proteins and fat; and proceed with detoxifying, neutralizing, and destroying substances such as drugs, pesticides, chemicals, and pollutants.

⚜ **They are therapeutic when administered for fatty liver, hepatitis, fibrosis, cirrhosis, and damage to the liver as the result of exposure to internal and environmental toxins.**

Dr. Benedikt suggests that for those with advanced liver pathology, the usual orthomolecular nutritional treatment protocols such as vitamin C, alpha-lipoic acid, milk thistle, curcuminoids, dandelion, green tea, and so on are not enough. Live liver peptide growth factors do the job, especially in chronic illnesses.

The more aggressive and effective treatment is Natcell Liver, which helps the patient's liver regenerate. However, frozen liquid liver peptide live cell extract may not be suitable for pregnant or nursing woman or for children under twelve years of age.

NATCELL MESENCHYME: TRANSFORMS DAMAGED CELLS

There has been a lack of public studies on Mesenchyme, due to the continued controversy regarding its source, which are embryonic cells or stem cells. The established thinking was that only human stem cells could be effective on humans, but newer studies have shown successful outcomes with animal cells. Embryonic stem cells work by seeking out damaged cells and transforming them into healthy ones. They work especially well in the liver.

Some studies have suggested that if humans were to use Mesenchyme at the late stage of requiring a liver transplant, up to 50% of those transplants might be unnecessary or, at least, delayed. Consider how much better off we might be if we started using Mesenchyme earlier on in the healing process.

One important thing which I learned early on was that people who used Natcell Thymus, Liver Extract, and Mesenchyme did far better than those who used Natcell Thymus alone. At the time, I was not sure why. But as I talked to people and observed them, I was eventually able to see that this particular combination worked near miracles for most users. I could never have afforded this very expensive program myself, but I quickly learned that the people who did use all three items regained their health faster.

Back in 2002, I contacted the company and asked them to make Natcell TLM — Thymus, Liver, and Mesenchyme in one vial. This was a successful attempt to lower the cost of the product. Natcell TLM is terrific for hepatitis C, hepatitis B, and other health concerns.

Natcell Mesenchyme alone offers tremendous help for those suffering from Hepatitis C and multiple sclerosis (MS). Let it be known that on "60 Minutes", Feb. 27, 2010 they reported that people who sold mesenchyme are snake oil salesmen. I am an observer. This product works and it works well. If you suffer from MS, use Natcell Mesenchyme. I have clients who say that when they use Mesenchyme they get out of their wheelchairs, forget about their canes, and enjoy life again.

Tendon damage caused by antibiotics like Cipro and Levaquin can also be reversed using Natcell Mesenchyme. I have many clients doing this now. Although it can take years for full recovery, it is the only treatment available for this distasteful and crippling side effect of antibiotics. People who suffer from knee pain and those who have had several surgeries have found relief with Natcell Mesenchyme.

NATCELL ADRENAL: ADRENAL GLAND SUPPORT

To support the adrenal glands, victims of hepatitis C should use Natcell Adrenal. Both hepatitis C and cancer patients can experience a significant improvement in their health by taking Natcell Adrenal, a live peptide. Adrenal gland supplements help the adrenal gland rebuild itself and improve overall liver function.

Adrenal glands are triangle-shaped glands located on top of the kidneys and they produce stress hormones. The outer part of the adrenal gland is called the cortex and it produces steroid hormones such as *cortisol, aldosterone,* and *testosterone.* The inner part of the adrenal gland is called the medulla and produces *epinephrine* and *norepinephrine,* which are commonly called adrenaline and noradrenaline.

When your adrenal glands produce more or less hormones than your body needs, you can become sick. Long-term stress, disease, radiation therapy and chemotherapy (including use of interferon) can damage the adrenal gland's medulla and cortex. When this occurs, disease begins to spread.

Physical exhaustion, demanding deadlines, infection, prolonged exposure to extreme temperatures, and major surgery all create stress. Stress puts intense pressure on the outer covering of adrenal glands, discharging high levels of hormones which helps the body's ability to survive stressful events. Producing adrenal hormones helps the organism survive stressful situations, but high levels of stress tax the adrenal glands and the immune system, and may diminish its efficiency and contribute to organ damage.

Working in conjunction with the adrenal gland, the liver displays extraordinary powers of regeneration after injury and during and after viral attack. An article published by Yale Medical School entitled, "Do Natural T Cells Promote Liver Regeneration," emphasizes the important of natural killer T cells in the regeneration of the liver.

During my treatment, I took two 300 mg. adrenal organic capsules a day. I suggest taking Natcell Adrenal, the finest adrenal supplement on earth, two vials a week or more. Because of its extreme expense I developed another product called Power Solution, an adrenal support product that is designed to be taken every day. Natcell Adrenal and Power Solution are also excellent choices to treat chronic fatigue.

How to Use the Frozen Liquid Porcine Peptide Growth Factors

1. *Peptides should be taken on an empty stomach in the morning or evening, half an hour before or two hours after a meal. Caution: NatCell Adrenal may cause sleep problems, take when your energy is low.*

2. *Thaw the 7 ml. vial of frozen liquid by holding in the hand.*

3. *Pour half of the vial's 7 ml. content (3.5 ml) under the tongue. Hold for five minutes, then swallow.*

4. *Repeat with second half of liquid.*

5. *Keep vial closed between steps.*

6. *Use as a nutritional supplement at the rate of two vials per week or more.*

SUPPLEMENTS AND HERBS

Basic supplements and herbs used in my program include milk thistle, alpha-lipoic acid, Reishi mushrooms, licorice root, dandelion, aloe vera, Vitamin C, olive leaf, NADH, cat's claw, Eurocel, Lipotrope, IP-6, Vitamin K2, and a good green super food.

Omega-3 supplements, and Vitamin D can be helpful if used judiciously. Burdock and hyssop are two particularly useful herb teas.

MILK THISTLE: ANCIENT BLESSING

Milk thistle is one of the oldest known medicinal herbs used to protect and strengthen the liver. Its main ingredient, silymarin, is widely available in capsule form. I also recommend drinking milk thistle tea.

Milk thistle strengthens liver cell walls, making it possible for toxins and poison to pass through the liver without causing damage. Milk thistle is foremost in healing chronic and acute liver damage.

I've reviewed many articles and studies on milk thistle and hope that some of them will find their way to all those liver doctors who told me there was nothing I could do or take to help my liver regenerate. Also modern-day liver doctors are always saying there are no studies on milk thistle.

Jean Rohrer comments:

"There has been recent clinical research, especially in Germany, which has brought the use of this multifunctional plant to front row prominence in the treatment of liver toxicity. Indeed, milk thistle is considered supreme in healing chronic or acute liver damage, virtually regardless of cause, as well as protecting the liver against many toxins and pollutants.

First, silymarin stabilizes and strengthens liver cell walls, stopping toxins from entering. It acts by inducing formation of liver cell proteins, which are incorporated into the cell walls, making them stronger and more resistant to toxins.

Second, by increasing the rate of protein synthesis, silymarin enhances regeneration of liver cells.

Third, are the antioxidants and free-radical scavenging abilities of this marvelous plant. As if these impressive effects weren't sufficient, the fourth mechanism silymarin gets involved in is the enzyme and catalytic activity of the liver. It inhibits production of the enzymes that produce substances damaging to the liver, while at the same time preventing the depletion of glutathione on liver cells, a substance that mediates cell metabolism.

Clinically, milk thistle causes significant reversal of symptoms of both acute and chronic liver problems from viral hepatitis to cirrhosis. [3]

During my treatment, I took two 400 mg. milk thistle capsules three times per day. I Also I drank one quart of milk thistle tea per day.

I recommend the tea because there are other active ingredients in milk thistle that are important, but unfortunately most of them are eliminated from the processed capsule form. Further, silymarin is not water soluble so it is important to use both capsules and drink the tea to get the most from milk thistle.

I use the organic milk thistle seeds, simmer them for one hour, and then drink the tea iced. I suggest 4 cups a day. Here is how to make it:

1. *Fill a 2-qt. pan with water.*

2. *Cover, bring to boil.*

3. *Rinse 1/2 cup milk thistle seeds.*

4. *Add milk thistle to boiling water.*

5. *Turn down heat to lowest flame, and cover.*

6. *Simmer (barely boiling) for one hour.*

7. *Add water as it evaporates to keep liquid at 2-qt. level.*

8. *Pour tea through strainer into container. Dilute to taste.*

9. *Cool, refrigerate, and enjoy. (Once it cools, it has a milky appearance.)*

ALPHA-LIPOIC ACID:
A POWERFUL ANTIOXIDANT

An antioxidant used in Europe to restore liver health, alpha-lipoic acid or ALA protects against oxidative processes involved in degenerative diseases. According to Dr. Ester Packer, professor of molecular biology at UC Berkeley, alpha-lipoic acid may be the most important antioxidant ever discovered. It is more potent antioxidant than vitamins C, E, and Coenzyme Q10, she says.

Alpha-lipoic acid occurs naturally in potatoes, sweet potatoes, carrots, yams, and red meat. But I take additional alpha-lipoic acid every day, and I know it has been vital in my conquest of hepatitis C.

During my treatment, I took two 100 mg. ALA capsules two times a day. Today, I suggest taking one 300 mg. capsule two times a day.

REISHI MUSHROOMS: ANCIENT REMEDY

For thousands of years, reishi mushrooms have been used in the Far East to promote good health.

According to David Law, the reishi mushroom is capable of increasing production of interleukin 1 and 2, known to inhibit tumor growth. Reishi mushrooms also have analgesic, anti-inflammatory, antioxidant, and anti-viral effects (through increased interferon production). Reishi mushrooms tend to lower blood pressure and act as a cardiovascular tonic by lowering serum cholesterol, and can provide liver protection and detoxification. Reishi mushrooms also protect against ionizing radiation and provide antibacterial and anti-HIV activity. [4]

Many studies show that immune boosting, antiviral reishi can dissolve tumor cells. A recent study by Cedars-Sinai Medical Center in Los Angeles, California shows that reishi can destroy primary liver cancer cells (hepatocellular carcinoma), a growing problem in the hepatitis C community. However, reishi should not be used as a stand-alone remedy for cancer.

During my treatment, I drank two cups of reishi tea each day, which is what I suggest. As an alternative, you may also take one 500 mg. reishi capsule three times a day. Suggested use is 2 cups of tea per day. Here's how to make the tea:

1. *Place 8 Reishi slices in 8 cups water.*

2. *Let soak overnight.*

3. *Next morning, simmer 45 minutes.*

4. *Remove from heat and drink, hot or cold.*

Important: Use only a glass teapot to brew Reishi tea!

LICORICE ROOT: BIOLOGICALLY ACTIVE

Licorice is one of the most biologically active herbs on earth. In Chinese medicine, licorice root is often used as a remedy for jaundice. It is considered a great liver detoxifier.

The licorice root derivatives such as glycyrrhetinic acid or GLA have proven extremely promising. Because licorice root increases the liver's ability to filter out toxins and waste products, it has proven extremely promising in the treatment of hepatitis and cirrhosis.

According to health writer Dan Mowrey, "experimental work has validated the usefulness of licorice in the treatment of hepatitis, cirrhosis, and related liver disorders." [5]

According to Mowrey, licorice root also helps prevent and heal skin problems, including eczema, dermatitis, impetigo, and traumatized skin. It helps reduce fever, which is common in people with hepatitis C. *However, if you have high blood pressure, do **not** use licorice root.*

During my treatment, I took one 500 mg. licorice root capsule two times a day, five days a week.

You might also try licorice root tea. And because licorice is 300 times sweeter than sugar, it makes an excellent sweetener of other teas. Suggested use is 1 or 2 cups a few days a week.

Here's how to make it:

1. *Fill a 2-qt. pan with water.*

2. *Cover, bring to a boil.*

3. *Add ½ cup licorice to boiling water, cover, and remove from heat.*

4. *Pour tea through a strainer into a container.*

5. *Cool, refrigerate and enjoy!*

DANDELION ROOT: A NATURAL LIVER TONIC

First mentioned as a medicinal plant by Arabian physicians of the 10th and 11th centuries, dandelion root is used today as a detoxifier for liver disease.

While undergoing radiation therapy for cancer, as my liver count test results soared, I recalled that my mother had always touted the benefits of dandelions for the liver. I began drinking two quarts of dandelion tea a day. After one month of adhering to that regimen, my ALT count dropped fifty points. Since then, I've been drinking dandelion root tea weekly.

In compromised liver conditions such as fibrosis and cirrhosis, the liver becomes less able to remove toxins from the blood and the liver itself becomes toxic. These toxins travel in the blood, and are able to cross the blood brain barrier, which can lead to brain fog and confusion. Dandelion helps remove these toxins, reduces brain fog, and cleans the liver, allowing us to live well. Dandelion also is a healthful diuretic that recent studies show is an excellent way to lower blood pressure.

During my treatment, I took one 500 mg. organic dandelion root capsule three times a day. I also made dandelion root tea and drank several cups every day. I suggest 4 cups a day or more, made like this:

1. *Fill a 2 quart pan with water.*
2. *Cover, bring to boil.*
3. *Rinse 1/2 cup dandelion root.*
4. *Add dandelion root to boiling water, and cover.*
5. *Remove from heat, and let brew for 1 hour.*
6. *Pour tea through a strainer into a container.*
7. *Dilute to taste. Can make 2-4 quarts. Cool, refrigerate, and enjoy.*

Note: You may mix in a dash of licorice to sweeten.

ALOE VERA:
HOLISTICALLY PERFECT PLANT

According to naturopath and author Dr. John Finnegan, the mucopolysaccharides found in aloe vera are also made in the human body and perform many key functions in our health, including growth and immune system functioning. Unfortunately, he says, after puberty our bodies stop manufacturing mucopolysaccharides and we must obtain them from outside sources.

Among a myriad of benefits, mucopolysaccharides: 1) make cells more resistant to virus and pathogenic bacteria; 2) improve overall cellular metabolism and functioning; 3) have anti-inflammatory properties; 4) provide critical lubrication of joints; help prevent and heal arthritis; 5) aid in absorption of water, minerals, and nutrients in the GI tract; 6) improve macrophage (white blood cells) activity, making them up to ten times more effective in engulfing foreign matter; 7) enhance the macrophage's effectiveness in modulating the entire immune system; 8) enhance the macrophage's ability to stimulate and direct the production and release of antibodies (increasing the body's own production of interferon, interleukins, and more; 9) increase the number of antibody forming T cells in the spleen and increase the number and activity of killer T-cell and monocyte activity; 10) are responsible for aloe vera's special penetration properties; 11) improve allergic reactions in conjunction with their cellular detoxification support and immune enhancement; 12) stimulate bone marrow activity; 13) stimulate the fibroblasts to release collagen and elastin to make new tissue (inside and out); 14) enhance immune system function and repair and detoxify the digestive and elimination systems of the body. [6]

Aloe vera supports the health and healing mechanisms of the body because it doesn't merely heal, it FEEDS THE BODY'S OWN SYSTEMS in order for them to function optimally, as they were originally designed to do.

The caveat here is that for an aloe vera product to be optimally effective, heat above 90°F must never be applied during processing, and it must never have been concentrated or diluted. The whole leaf must be used, as it is more potent in that form, but the substance aloin—which can irritate the bowel—should be completely removed or lowered to a concentration of 1 part per million or less. There is only one whole leaf aloe vera product sold in the U.S. that I know is non-pasteurized—Herbal Aloe Force.

During my treatment, I drank four ounces of properly prepared (see above paragraph) aloe vera two to four times a day, usually more often.

VITAMIN C: WONDER NUTRIENT

Vitamin C is a true wonder nutrient which has a lot of health benefits. During my treatment, I took 7,000 mg. of vitamin C a day for three months.

According to Hans Larsen, author of *Vitamin C: Your Ultimate Health Insurance*, Vitamin C reduces the severity of a cold, effectively prevents secondary viral and bacterial complications, stimulates the immune system and protects against damage by the free radicals released into the body by infection. [7]

Larsen contends that a daily intake of 250-1,000 mg. of vitamin C may act as a preventative measure, but he believes that far larger quantities are required to halt or reverse cancer, heart disease, and hepatitis C.

In order to get sufficient vitamin C in my diet, I consumed at least two fresh lemons every day. They should be fresh and organic, and can easily be used in tea, marinated meat, stir-fry dishes, lemonade, lemon honey, and added to water. Lemons are a good source of magnesium, which helps maintain the body's mineral balance.

Lemons are an excellent natural source of Vitamin C. Renowned herbalist Maud Grieve said, "It is probable that the lemon is the most valuable of all fruits for preserving health." [8]

When dealing with hepatitis C, we need far more vitamin C than is found in food. Often doctors like to use IV drips of vitamin C. These are fine for many serious conditions and can help. They lower the viral load, AST and ALT in many cases. However when one stops the IV, the viral load, AST and ALT go right back where they were.

I have found that Ultra Absorbic C, a liquid vitamin C that incorporates Ethanol and EDTA for absorption through the colon wall gets 90% of the Vitamin C into your blood while the normal vitamin C supplements get less than 10% into your blood. I have observed thousands of clients who have used this vitamin C since 2002 and I can say over time it provides a better outcome than IV drip.

OLIVE LEAF:
NATURE'S ANTIVIRAL

The key antiviral and antibacterial agent in olive leaf extract is oleuropein. This increases blood flow in coronary arteries, relieves arrhythmias, and prevents intestinal muscle spasms which are important in treating hepatitis C.

According to James R. Privitera, M.D., some unique properties of olive leaf are: 1) interference with critical amino acid production essential for virus survival; 2) containment of viral infection by inactivating viruses or preventing virus shedding, budding, or assembly at cell membrane; 3) penetration of infected cells to stop viral replication; 4) neutralization of transcriptase (a protease) production—essential for enabling retroviruses like HIV to alter the RNA of a healthy cell; and 5) stimulation of phagocytosis, an immune system response wherein cells ingest harmful microorganisms and foreign matter (bacteria and viruses.)

In addition to hepatitis B and C, olive leaf extract is effective against herpes, flu and colds, bacterial infections, diabetes, rheumatoid arthritis, chronic fatigue syndrome, allergies, vaginal yeast infections, skin conditions, and malaria. Recent studies also indicate that olive leaf can be an effective treatment for high blood pressure.

During my treatment, I took one 500 mg. of olive leaf extract capsule three days a week.

NADH: SYNERGIZE YOUR NEUROTRANSMITTERS

Nicotinamide Adenine Dinucleotide or NADH is an enzyme which is directly involved in the cellular immune defense system. It reduces ferric iron and strengthens blood hemoglobin.

Within the body, special white blood cells called macrophages are responsible for the elimination of foreign bodies such as bacteria, viruses, and molds. NADH literally captures these foreign bodies and degrades and eliminates them through a phenomenon known as "metabolic burst." This appears to be the first and most critical step toward the ultimate destruction of foreign invaders by the immune system.

Present in all living cells, NADH is found in greatest abundance in meat, fish, and chicken. Since food preparation destroys most of it, and the digestive process destroys more, it is helpful to use NADH supplements in the treatment of hepatitis C.

A crucial antioxidant, NADH protects the body from free radicals and the ravages of aging. It also enhances the capacity of your immune system and protects cells from damage by toxins and environmental pollution.

NADH increases brain functions and cognitive

capabilities, protects the liver from alcohol damage, prevents alcohol-induced inhibition of testosterone biosynthesis, normalizes cholesterol levels and blood pressure, and offers protection from certain toxins, such as the AIDS drug AZT and other carcinogens without depleting the positive effects of the drug.

"NADH is required for synthesis of neurotransmitters, which explains its effect on maintaining healthy mind and mental functions. NADH is the co-enzymatic form of vitamin B-3. NADH is involved in production of energy in all cells."

In the brain, messages received from the body are transmitted between approximately fifteen billion brain cells by chemicals called neurotransmitters. For those who have used interferon, this communication is often disrupted, creating what is sometimes called "brain fog."

In my case, at one point interferon devastated these transmissions so much that I was unable to draw a simple line between numbers on a test by a state-appointed neurologist/psychiatrist. This person explained that my use of interferon resulted in symptoms similar to those of Gulf War Syndrome. NADH is also very good for Chronic Fatigue.

During my treatment, I took one 5 mg. tablet of NADH each morning on an empty stomach.

CAT'S CLAW:
IMMUNE BOOSTER

Cat's claw or *uncaria tamentosa* grows in the rainforest of the Peruvian Amazon, where it's been used as a medicinal plant since the time of the ancient Incas. Cat's claw tea is known for arresting and reversing deep-seated pathologies in the body. The inner bark has unique active constituents that help support the body's natural defenses.

Six oxindole alkaloids have been isolated from cat claw's inner bark. These have been proven to provide a general boost to the immune system and a profound effect on the ability of white blood cells to engulf and digest harmful microorganisms and foreign matter. Other alkaloids and phytochemicals present in the herb have been proven useful against many viruses and explain its antioxidant, antibacterial, anti-tumor, and anti-inflammatory properties.

During my treatment, I took two 500 mg. cat's claw capsules two times a day. I also drank two cups of cat's claw tea a day.

Because it may cause drowsiness, it is also a useful bedtime beverage. I suggest 1 or 2 cups a few days a week.

To make the tea, mix one teaspoon of cat's claw powder into one cup of hot water.

EUROCEL:
THREE ANCIENT HERBS

Eurocel is a product made from three medicinal herbs that have been used for years in Oriental medicine — *Patrinia villosa, Artemisla capollaris,* and *Schizandra fructus.*

During a pilot study of 10 patients with hepatitis C in which all ten patients responded well, 2 mg. of this herbal combination were taken twice daily. Elevated liver enzyme levels, indicators of liver damage, dropped to normal levels, and hepatitis C virus RNA levels gradually became lower over the course of therapy. After twenty-four months of taking the herbs, some subjects' viral titer count decreased from levels measures in the millions to levels in the thousands, a drop of up to one million-fold. ALT, bilirubin, albumin, total protein, and cholesterol levels also improved.

Better quality of sleep, increased physical energy, increased body weight, and smoother, softer skin were immediately reported by a majority of subjects. No adverse symptoms were reported.

I suggest two capsules of Eurocel three times a day on an empty stomach.

LIPOTROPE:
HELP FOR A FATTY LIVER

The liver removes fatty acids from food or accumulated fat deposits by degrading and oxidizing them when the body must call on fat as a major energy source. Lipotropic factors, a key to this process, must be active to prevent abnormal accumulation of fats in the liver. By a process called transmethylation, lipotropic agents promote the production of lipoproteins, which transfer fatty acids out of the liver. [9]

Lipotrope prevents fat accumulation in the liver. Lipotrope also aids a vital process called hormone conjugation. Calcium, protein, mineral, and fat metabolism are all regulated by components of conjugated estrogen. Without this process, hormones such as estrogen can become carcinogenic.

A normal liver fat is about 5-15% fat, whereas a diabetic's liver is 25-35% fat. The percentage of fat in the liver increases with excessive alcohol consumption, the use of birth control pills, estrogen usage, high vitamin B-1 and B12 intake, and cobalt treatments.

Among other conditions, liver dysfunction causes fatigue, constipation, hypertension, glaucoma, blood sugar metabolic imbalance, arteriosclerosis, hepatitis, and jaundice.

During my treatment, I took one Lipotrope capsules three times a day.

INOSITOL HEXAPHOSPHATE: IP-6 HELPS LOWER FERRITIN

Inositol and its derivative inositol hexaphosphate or IP-6 are ever present in most plant and animal cells. IP-6 can help lower ferritin or iron in the liver. IP-6 has been shown in hundreds of studies to also be very effective in fighting many types of cancer.

While approximately 30% of people with hepatitis C have high ferritin, doctors have no idea what it is and less of a clue about treating it. High ferritin causes serious symptoms in most cases, fatigue being the most prominent. High ferritin also raises the AST and ALT.

IP-6 is slow and inefficient. A therapeutic phlebotomy (the removal of about a pint of blood) is the quickest and best way to lower your ferritin level. However, often the hepatitis C patient has low platelets and a therapeutic phlebotomy cannot be done. This is when one uses IP-6.

The amount needed varies from person to person, from one to six capsules at a time, two to four times per day. Take IP-6 with water on an empty stomach—no food for 40 minutes before and after.

VITAMIN K2:
MAY PREVENT LIVER CANCER

Studies show that Vitamin K2 can help prevent up to 80% of primary liver cancer caused by cirrhosis. If you have hepatitis C, consider yourself a candidate for cirrhosis at some point.

Primary liver cancer can take years to develop. Most cases are treatable. Start taking Vitamin K2 now.

When researchers in the Graduate School of Medicine of Japan's Osaka City University began studying vitamin K on a group of women with cirrhosis of the liver, their goal was to evaluate the potential of using vitamin K to prevent bone loss. But the final analysis of data revealed an unexpected benefit, as reported in *The Journal of the American Medical Association.*

The Osaka team recruited 40 women with viral cirrhosis and most of the subjects also had hepatitis C. The average age for the group was about 60. For two years, 21 subjects took a daily 45 mg dose of vitamin K2. The other 19 women took a placebo. Of the women who took K2 group, only two developed liver cancer, while nine of the women in the placebo group developed cancer.

The study also found that vitamin K2 supplementation helped prevent bone loss in women with cirrhosis of the liver.

TWO HELPFUL HERB TEAS:

HYSSOP TEA can cleanse the system, provide energy and promote a vibrantly healthy attitude. Hyssop is a remarkable herb and should be considered by everyone with hepatitis C.

Hyssop is mentioned more times in the Bible than any other herb. In the book of Genesis 1-30, God spoke of giving mankind herb-bearing seed, in Ezekiel 47-12 it is written, *"And the fruit thereof shall be meat, and the leaf thereof for medicine."*

In the first Passover described in the book of Exodus, Moses gave a detailed account of the rituals where hyssop was used as a cleansing herb to protect the household. The Bible also records that hyssop was used to clean lepers. Hippocrates used hyssop to treat pleurisy.

I suggest a hyssop tea cleanse once a month. Drink 2 quarts per day for 3 days; avoid meat & dairy during cleanse.

1. *Fill a 2-qt. pan with water.*
2. *Cover, bring to boil.*
3. *Add 1 cup hyssop to boiling water and cover.*
4. *Remove from heat, and let brew for 1 hour.*
5. *Pour tea through strainer into container.*
6. *Cool, refrigerate, and enjoy.*

BURDOCK TEA helps in treating indigestion, strengthening and toning the stomach, easing bladder pain, reducing fluid retention, and alleviating gout. It also helps in stimulating the eliminatory organs and treating glandular conditions, hepatitis and liver problems and reduces jaundice and inflammation! Suggested use: 1 cup 2 times a day

1. *Bring 2 quarts water to boil.*

2. *Add ½ cup burdock root, and cover.*

3. *Remove from heat, and let brew for one hour.*

BE VERY CAREFUL WITH:

OMEGA-3s:
EASY DOES IT

Omega-3 fatty acids are essential fatty acids. They are necessary for human health but the body can't make them — you have to get Omega-3s through food. Also known as polyunsaturated fatty acids, Omega-3 fatty acids play a crucial role in brain function as well as normal growth and development. They have also become popular because they may reduce the risk of heart disease.

Omega-3 fatty acids can be found in fish, such as salmon, tuna, halibut, and krill, other seafood including algae, and some plants, and nut oils.

Please take the standard suggested doses. A compromised liver has trouble with excessive amounts. There are many different types of omega 3 today and most of them are made from mixed fish. Larger fish have far more mercury content and should be avoided. Use only omega 3 made from Krill, a very small fish which is low on the food chain.

VITAMIN D: DON'T OVERDO IT

Many benefits of Vitamin D have finally been discovered by health care practitioners and as a result high doses are being recommended. I see health care practitioners, naturopathic doctors, etc., prescribing 5,000-10,000 IU a day for their patients with hepatitis C. However, this much additional Vitamin D raises ALT and AST and can raise the viral load in chronic Hepatitis C. Stick with between 400 IU and 800 IU of Vitamin D. Also work on getting your D from full sun.

PROMISING NEW SUPPLEMENTS

In recent times, I have found a few exceptional supplements to add to my program. New studies show terrific benefits for naringenin, blueberry extract, oxymatrine, quercetin, zinc, catechin, cartilade, and lactoferrin

NARINGENIN: POWERFUL FLAVONOID

A powerful flavonoid found in grapefruit called naringenin shows promise in helping to combat hepatitis C.

The hepatitis C virus is bound to a very low intensity lipo-protein (one of the so-called "bad" cholesterols), when it is secreted from liver cells, according to a February 4, 2007, article published in *Science Daily*. Researchers at the Massachusetts General Hospital Center for Engineering in Medicine reported that the viral secretion required to pass infection to other cells may be blocked by the common flavonoid naringenin.

The Massachusetts experiments confirm that naringenin does reduce the secretion of the hepatitis C virus from infected liver cells and show that the compound inhibits the mechanism for secreting a specific lipoprotein that binds the HCV.

Naringenin can reduce a chronic infection to an acute infection. However, naringenin also slows the liver's ability to remove some drugs from the body. At least one half of my clients take too many prescription drugs to use this extremely beneficial supplement. On the other hand, I have had some clients who say they became non-detected using only naringenin. Caution: Do not take if you are taking high blood pressure medication.

BLUEBERRY EXTRACT: 45% PROANTHOCYANIDIN

Japanese researchers Hiroaki Kataoka and colleagues at the University of Miyazaki, Japan searched for agricultural products containing a natural agent to fight the Hepatitis C virus. They discovered that blueberry leaves contained a substance that inhibited the replication of the hepatitis C virus. Upon persistent purification and testing of their most effective hepatitis C-halting extract, the active ingredient was determined to be the antioxidant proanthocyanidin.

"Purified proanthocyanidin showed dose-dependent inhibition of expression of the neomycin-resistant gene and the NS-3 protein gene in the HCV subgenome in replicon cells. While characterizing the mechanism by which proanthocyanidin inhibited HCV subgenome expression, we found that heterogeneous nuclear ribonucleoprotein A2/B1 showed affinity to blueberry leaf-derived proanthocyanidin and was indispensable for HCV sub-genome expression in replicon cells. These data suggest that proanthocyanidin isolated from blueberry leaves may have potential usefulness as an anti-HCV compound by inhibiting viral replication," the authors reported in *The Journal of Biological Chemistry.*

I tried to find a product like this so I could provide it for the hepatitis C community, but could not, so I made my own. Each 300 mg capsule contains 45% proanthocyanidin. I have seen great success with Blueberry extract at lowering the AST, ALT and viral load. Also my clients see a reduction of overall symptoms and a healthier frame of mind. A side benefit is that some are experiencing better vision. I for one have taken my blueberry extract every day since I first made it and found that I no longer need to use reading glasses.

Take 2 caps in the AM and 2 caps in the PM.

OXYMATRINE: PROTECTIVE EFFECTS

Oxymatrine is one of the unique alkaloids present in sophora roots or *kushen* used in traditional Chinese medicine, where it is classed as a sedative. Oxymatrine has the ability to lower the viral load, AST, ALT, improve quality of sleep, reduce symptoms, and provide a better quality of life.

Among the earliest publications about clinical application of oxymatrine for viral hepatitis was a preliminary study by Li Jiqiang and colleagues studying patients with hepatitis C. Their report claimed positive results. It was published in Chinese in 1998 and again in English in 1999.

The inhibitory effect of oxymatrine on hepatitis C virus was confirmed by Chen Yanxi and his colleagues at the Shanghai Second Medical University in cell culture tests. A protective effect of oxymatrine against liver cell death was indicated in a pharmacology study with non-viral (immune-based) liver damage.

These positive results led to a second, longer study, in which the researchers recruited 144 patients with either hepatitis B or hepatitis C. Patients were randomly separated into two groups: oxymatrine (group A) and placebo (group B). The patients took 900 mg capsules of oxymatrine every day for 52 weeks. The authors of the study concluded that oxymatrine could effectively treat chronic viral hepatitis and promote the serum markers of hepatitis B virus (HBV) and hepatitis C virus (HCV) in chronic hepatitis B and C to convert to negative and reduce serum level of ALT.

To evaluate further the mechanisms of oxymatrine in hepatitis patients, a study was set-up to test several additional blood parameters as affected by injection and capsule forms of oxymatrine. Serum cholinesterase and liver function tests improved, while other serum parameters such as albumin and prothrombin activity were unaffected. A laboratory investigation into the mechanism of oxymatrine suggested that there might also be an immune-based response to the virus involving the T-cells.

QUERCETIN:
NO CELL TOXICITY

Several laboratory studies show quercetin, a bioflavonoid found in plants, may have anti-inflammatory and antioxidant properties. Used by many people as a nutritional supplement, quercetin is currently being investigated for a wide range of potential health benefit.

At a 2011 medical conference, Samuel Wheeler French Jr., MD, PhD, Assistant Professor of Pathology and Laboratory Medicine at UCLA, reported that quercetin can help stop production of the hepatitis C virus without any cell toxicity.

ZINC:
IMPROVES LONG-TERM OUTCOMES

Zinc supplementation can improve the outcomes for chronic hepatitis C and liver cirrhosis, according to a study by Shunichi Matsuoka of the Division of Gastroenterology and Hepatology, Department of Medicine, Nihon University School of Medicine, in Tokyo. Dr. Matsuoka's study measured serum zinc concentrations using conventional atomic absorption spectrometry to determine the long-term outcome of zinc therapy.

Dr. Matsuoka reported that changes of AST and ALT levels in the zinc administration group were significantly lower than those of the untreated group. The decrease in platelet count was clearly less than that of the untreated group. When patients who were administered zinc were divided into two groups whose zinc concentrations increased (zinc responders) or remained stable or decreased (zinc non-responders), the zinc responders had a clearly lower cumulative incidence of liver cancer than the zinc non-responders. His study concluded that zinc supplementation improved long-term outcomes in people with hepatitis C and hepatocellular carcinoma.

CATECHIN:
POWERFUL ANTIVIRAL ACTIVITY

Scientists at the University of California at Los Angeles (UCLA) have discovered that a plant-derived bioflavonoid, catechin, displays powerful antiviral activity on tissue cultures infected with hepatitis C, according to an article in the online newspaper *Natural News*, on April 13, 2011. Catechin is found in abundance in green tea extract, and also in beans and chocolate.

CARTILADE:
HELPS JOINT PAIN

People with hepatitis C and people who have used interferon often have moderate to severe joint pain, chronic rheumatoid or osteoarthritis. There are many different supplements available but the one that I've found that's completely natural and effective is Cartilade.

Cartilade shark cartilage contains mucopolysaccharides, a family of complex carbohydrates including the now well-known chondroitin sulfate. It is an excellent source of calcium and phosphorus.

Cartilade contains 12% chondroitin, Type II collagen, 35% protein and 50% minerals essential for connective tissue synthesis. More importantly, Cartilade exhibits the highest rate of matrix metalloproteinases or MMP inhibition, and the highest inhibition of destructive catabolic activity of the connective tissues and joints. It is the only shark cartilage brand with this proven activity.

LACTOFERRIN: IMPROVES LIVER FUNCTION

Mayo Clinic infectious disease specialist James Steckelberg, M.D., states that a substance called lactoferrin may show promise for a treatment for hepatitis C. A few small studies suggest lactoferrin may reduce levels of the hepatitis C virus in the blood and improve liver function. Also, the combination of lactoferrin and Phosphatidyl Choline, another dietary supplement, has been shown to reduce liver enzymes.

What they did not say is that lactoferrin will raise the level of iron in your system. Fortunately there is one brand that has the iron removed, Apolactoferrin. I have been providing this for a few years and find that it reduces liver inflammation, relieves "baseball under the rib" syndrome, can lower the AST, ALT, and viral load.

Lysine

I have been providing lysine to a small group of clients. All of them have displayed reduced AST and ALT in the first few months. I will keep you informed on my investigation on lysine.

FOODS TO EAT,
FOODS TO AVOID

Certain foods can strengthen your liver and your body. On the other hand, a few common foods should be avoided by people with hepatitis C.

Generally speaking, hepatitis C patients should avoid overloading on meat protein, which can create a rise in ammonia levels that adversely affects the central nervous system. Avoid fast food, fried food, and fatty food. Steamed vegetables and grains, along with limited amounts of chicken, fish, and turkey are good sources for vitamins and protein. Bee pollen is also very good for high ammonia levels.

Especially good for rebuilding the liver are artichokes, buckwheat, and spinach, raw yogurt from good quality milk, avocados, and hot chocolate. Also good to include in your diet are beet tops, beets, lemons and lemon juice, carrots, greens, whole grains, organic liver, and egg yolks. However, pasteurized homogenized milk, hard liquor, hydrogenated oils, white sugar, white flour and a few other items should be avoided.

ARTICHOKES:
PROTECT THE LIVER

In 1969, French scientists were so successful in using artichoke extract for treating liver and kidney ailments, they took out a patent on it. In fact, cynarin, a constituent of the artichoke, was formulated into a drug to lower blood cholesterol. It is also a liver protective. [10]

Native to the Mediterranean, the artichoke is a perennial in the thistle group. Eat two a day, preferably organically grown, and wash thoroughly. Available in jars and cans, they make a great appetizer and are good in salads.

BUCKWHEAT:
RICH IN PHYTONUTRIENTS

Widely recognized as a liver cleanser, buckwheat flour can be substituted for conventional wheat flour as it does not contain gluten. Buckwheat's beneficial effects are due in part to its rich supply of flavonoids, particularly *rutin*. One type of phytonutrients especially abundant in whole grains such as buckwheat are plant lignans, which are converted by friendly flora in our intestines into mammalian lignans, including one thought to protect against certain cancers as well as heart disease. Flavonoids protect against disease by extending the action of vitamin C and acting as antioxidants.

Health food stores carry cereals and noodles made from buckwheat, which is also high in insoluble fiber. Buckwheat flour can be mixed with whole wheat flour to make delicious breads, muffins and pancakes. A pot of cooked buckwheat can be a breakfast substitute for oatmeal. You can also add cooked buckwheat to soups or stews to give them a heartier flavor and deeper texture.

SPINACH:
HIGH IN CAROTENOIDS

Consistently rated high in surveys as a strong cancer preventive, several studies have found that spinach may help prevent liver cancer.

According to best-selling health book author Jean Carper, an analysis by the United States Department of Agriculture revealed that raw spinach contains a very high level (36 milligrams) of total carotenoids per hundred grams, whereas raw carrots have only 14 milligrams per hundred grams, mostly attributable to beta-carotene.

YOGURT: SUPER IMMUNE BOOSTER

Yogurt contains beneficial bacteria which help digestion and strengthen the body.

"Benefits of Yogurt," a report published in the *Journal of Immunotherapy*, reveals that yogurt-based *acidophilus*, when eaten over a period of several months, increased natural gamma-inter-feron, an immune-enhancing protein that prevents viruses from reproducing, and reduced inflammatory responses of the gut. Additionally, IgE, an immunoglobulin effective in destroying parasites, is enhanced when *lactobacillus bulgaricus* found in yogurt is added to the diet. [11]

According to Khem Shahani, PhD., an author who has done research on probiotics, *lactobacillus acidophilus,* one of the beneficial bacteria in yogurt: 1) enhances the immune system by eliminating or inhibiting the formation of cancer-causing chemicals, 2) halts the conversion of nitrates into carcinogenic nitrosamines in the gut by reducing the quantity of potential carcinogens, and by deactivating certain cancer-causing enzymes, especially d-glucrondase and b-glocosidase.

I consumed raw yogurt daily during my recovery period, and still do.

AVOCADOS:
MAY REDUCE LIVER DAMAGE

Researchers in Japan have discovered that avocados contain potent chemicals that may reduce liver damage.

Five compounds appear to be active in creating the fruit's benefits. Each was tested in rats with chemically induced liver injuries resembling those caused by viruses. This suggests that avocados may be especially promising for the treatment of viral hepatitis, according to the International Chemical Congress of Pacific Basin Societies.

I created and lived on an avocado farm from 1980 until 1987. During this time, I consumed a great number of avocados. I still do, and I suggest you do the same. Enjoy them in salads, sandwiches, guacamole or plain. They taste delicious, and are good for your liver.

HOT CHOCOLATE: GOOD FOR THE BODY

According to research presented on April 15, 2010, to the International Live Congress in Austria, consumption of dark chocolate could be used to aid patients suffering from cirrhosis of the liver and those who have high blood pressure in the abdomen.

The study showed a clear association between dark chocolate and **portal hypertension,** and demonstrated the potential importance of improvements in the management of people with cirrhosis, to minimize the onset and impact of end-stage liver disease and its associated mortality risks.

This study adds to an ever-growing body of science supporting the health benefits of consuming cocoa flavonoids.

The last two words in my very first book, published in June 1999 were: "Eat Chocolate."

FOOD ITEMS TO AVOID:

AVOID HOMOGENIZED, PASTEURIZED DAIRY PRODUCTS

Milk is naturally produced by mothers for the nourishment of their young. Nourishing milk in the form of colostrum is produced by mothers to nourish newborn children. Milk contains many essential nutrients, enzymes, and other factors that are destroyed by heat.

Milk is pasteurized by heating it to a high temperature for a period of time to kill bacteria. This heating process also destroys most of the essential elements of milk, making it relatively worthless to consume.

All milk products are also homogenized, including cheese and sour cream, etc. The homogenization of milk blends small droplets of butter fat into the milk and causes an impaired liver to work harder to deal with this processed food.

Pasteurized, homogenized milk is a completely unnatural food that the human body has never had to deal with until the twentieth century. Dr. Kurt Oster and many other physicians consider homogenized milk the number one cause of heart disease in the United States. [12]

Raw milk and products made from raw milk are safe and healthy alternatives when available.

Considering the quality of milk available in the modern world, you might consider supplementing with colostrum, which is milk taken from a mammal, usually a cow, from the time they give birth until approximately eighteen hours later. An essential immune booster, colostrum is filled with many wonder-nutrients unavailable in any other product.

AVOID HYDROGENATED OIL

Dr. John Finnegan warns that more than 200 million people may have been killed by the combined harmful effects of refined oils and deficiencies of Omega-3 fatty acids. This exceeds the total number of fatalities in all the wars of the 20th century.

Dr. Finnegan says it takes six to nine months for hydrogenated oil to pass through the liver, where it acts as a poisonous agent.

AVOID HARD LIQUOR

Hard liquor is hard on your liver. If you are a drinker, your probability of receiving a liver transplant—should it become a necessity—is slim to none. Because liquor inflames the liver, for those of you with hepatitis C, it will likely make you feel sicker and this will only take the fun out of drinking. It's best to minimize your alcohol intake, or reduce it to zero.

AVOID SUGAR SUBSTITUTES (SACCHARINE, EQUAL, ETC.)

It is my understanding that sugar substitutes, especially saccharine, require sixty times more effort by the liver to process than sugar. Furthermore, their labels clearly warn of the cancer risk. My recommendation is to use honey and raw sugar instead.

AVOID REFINED SUGAR, WHITE FLOUR, SALT

Start preventing additional health problems now. Avoid white refined sugar, white flour, and salt. Refined sugar and white flour have almost no nutrients. Do not eat salt because it makes fibrosis and cirrhosis worse. Most packaged or canned goods contain salt. Find products labeled "no salt added" or "low sodium." **Salt kills in cirrhosis.**

AVOID VITAMIN E & RESVERATROL

The Department of Internal Medicine at the Keio University Medical School in Tokyo on Jan. 14, 2010 provided research that shows that resveratrol raises the viral load in HCV and that Vitamin E also raises the viral load.

If you are going to take Vitamin E, take the water soluble product Vitamin E succinate. The oil based product available in health food stores also raises the AST and ALT.

A HEALTHY LIFESTYLE

A lifestyle that promotes good health for people with hepatitis C involves more than good nutrition and supplements. It includes practicing personal cleanliness, avoiding excessive stress, exercising regularly, and having a good spiritual relationship with your God.

PERSONAL CLEANLINESS

Albumin is a protein made in the liver and found in the blood and body tissues. Albumin is involved in just about everything your body does. According to scientist Kenneth Seeton, a person's albumin count is the prime factor in determining health. Practicing cleanliness can keep your albumin level closer to optimum levels, and help you deal with hepatitis C.

In the Old Testament, God spoke to Moses and Aaron. God prescribed detailed methods for cleansing the body and washing cloths properly under circumstances such as handling the dead and preventing the spread of disease. God's recommendations involved cleansing the body using water, various herbs such as hyssop, and allowing adequate drying time. We know now that these instructions helped prevent the spread of disease and the transmission of bacteria and viruses from person to person.

As usual, medical science was slow to get the message. In the 1840s, a young European doctor named Ignay Semmelweis discovered that ordering hospital doctors wash their hands after doing autopsies or before examining each patients resulted in miraculously low mortality rates in obstetrical wards. For his discovery, Semmelweis was dismissed from the hospital and horribly persecuted for what has now become standard good medical practice.

A low albumin count is directly related to liver disease. The balance of albumin should be at least 4.8 grams per liter. The average in the U.S. is only 4.1. When your albumin falls below 3, life becomes precious.

Your albumin count cannot be raised by diet. That albumin count is connected to cleanliness—which is next to godliness – is a proven fact. However, every single medical doctor I have mentioned this to has come back with an arrogant response.

The immune system can be overloaded with bacteria and viruses, and weakened by producing antibodies to battle them. This accounts for many viral load spikes which can send patients into a debilitating panic when they show up on medical tests.

Kenneth Seeton believes that 80% of all disease is transmitted to ourselves through rubbing of the eyes and nose. The only way to bring the antibodies down is by removing the possibility of infection from eyes and nose.

This can be done, as God told Moses long ago, by practicing personal cleanliness. One way to lower the overload on the immune system is to wash your hands and fingernails four to twenty times a day. In addition, drinking adequate water every day also prevents dehydration, which adversely affects albumin levels.

If you wish to overcome Hepatitis C, it is critical to follow the previous scenario absolutely in order to free up the immune system and boost it in order to conquer your potentially fatal disease.

MINIMIZE STRESS

Livers don't like stress. Stress breaks down the immune system. The body is not designed to deal with stress except in the short term.

It is hard to avoid stress, especially when your doctor has just advised you that you have hepatitis C and that you are going to die a horrible death. You give up hope for a liver transplant when you learn that for every one person who receives one, many patients die waiting. Ultimately, the doctor will send you off with a prescription for interferon, which can negatively impact your behavior. What are your chances for avoiding stress in this stark scenario?

Find an outlet that will help you relieve that tension. Exercise. Read and re-read this book. Consult a spiritual advisor. Pray. Meditate. Do something you've always wanted to do and haven't yet done. Go to a concert, a play, a sporting event. Fly a kite, take a trip, confess your love to someone dear to you. And, of course, eat chocolate! It's a mild mood elevator, and a good antioxidant.

EXERCISE

Exercise helps every part of the body work as it should, since the human body was designed to move frequently. Exercise helps the body expel toxins. I recommend daily exercise, as much as possible given one's physical limitations. Exercise is not only a stress-buster, it also stimulates circulation of the lymph, which is part of the body's natural immune system. Exercise helps the heart pump oxygen-rich blood from the lungs all through the body and vital organs.

Chapter 4

SPECIAL
HEALTH ISSUES

This chapter looks at special health issues of interest. Certain vaccinations and pharmaceutical drugs, for instance, should definitely be avoided.

Over time, people with hepatitis C develop fibrosis which can lead to cirrhosis of the liver. Serious complications of liver disease that may occur include portal hypertension, varices, ascites and liver cancer. Fortunately, there are hopeful new medical developments on the horizon.

HEPATITIS A & B VACCINES

When one is first diagnosed with hepatitis C, one of the most common things to happen is your doctor will automatically give you the hepatitis A & B vaccine. Most medical doctors will cause one to believe that this is mandatory and often just give people the first shot. If one objects, they are often subjected to a surprising amount of ridicule and harassment. One client told me her doctor said, "Why are you afraid? My 6-year old son just had it."

Let me say that people with hepatitis C have a completely different reaction to the A & B vaccine than healthy people. This first period of time is often the beginning of the domino effect in health and hepatitis C.

After receiving these vaccines, your viral load is going to go up millions of points and it will take nine months to two years before it starts to come back down. Your AST and ALT are going to go up for a time. Prior to 2002, these vaccines were not distributed the way they are now.

In 1999, my client Jenny was working very diligently on getting well. She started with a viral load of a little over seven million and got it down to 36,000 in one year. She was working hard at this. She even went to a school to learn about natural medicine, ate right, took all the right supplements, and was very enthusiastic about her progress. Then her doctor told her, run, don't walk, to the clinic to get your hepatitis A & B vaccine. Her viral load shot up to 17,000,000, and her AST and ALT jumped into the hundreds. Jenny was devastated, and I did not hear from her for many months. Then one day I saw her, and she told me what had happened, that she had worked so hard over such a long time, was very diligent in everything she did, and then one day after taking the A & B vaccine, her viral load was over 17,000,000. I then explained to her that I observe this all the time. Jenny thought that her program had simply failed, but it was the medical community's mistake that led to her downfall, not the failure of her program. We then worked together on getting her viral load down again, and we did manage to get it to 7,000,000 and restore her health and attitude, and got her back on track.

It is important to understand that if you have hepatitis C and you contract hepatitis A, you are going to get sick and may die. If you live in the United States, however, a person with hepatitis C is more likely to be hit by a bolt of lightning than to contract the hepatitis A virus. If you are planning on traveling to a destination where hepatitis A is epidemic, I suggest you change your travel plans.

If you have hepatitis C and contract hepatitis B, you can live with only minor complications as long as your liver is in good shape. If you have C and took the vaccines, do the best you can. It just takes longer.

One more reason I do not recommend the hepatitis B vaccine is this information about the relationship of the hepatitis B virus and liver cancer, quoted here from *www.Medicinenet.com:*

"The most convincing reason comes from a prospective (looking forward in time) study done in the 1970s in Taiwan, involving male government employees over the age of 40. In this study, the investigators found that the risk of developing liver cancer was 200 times higher among employees who had chronic hepatitis B virus.

"Studies in animals also have provided evidence that hepatitis B virus can cause liver cancer. For example, we have learned that liver cancer develops in other mammals that are naturally infected with viruses related to the hepatitis B virus. Finally by infecting transgenic mice with certain parts of the hepatitis B virus, scientists caused liver cancer to develop in mice that do not usually develop liver cancer. [Transgenic mice are mice that have been injected with new or foreign genetic material.]

"How does chronic hepatitis B virus cause liver

cancer? In patients with both chronic hepatitis B virus and liver cancer, the genetic material of hepatitis B virus is frequently found to be part of the genetic material of the cancer cells. It is thought therefore, that specific regions of the hepatitis B virus genome (genetic code) enter the genetic material of the liver cells. This hepatitis B virus genetic material may then disrupt the normal genetic material in the liver cells, thereby causing the liver cells to become cancerous."

Considering this and the fact that the B vaccine can get into the genetic code and possibly cause liver cancer in a compromised liver is enough for me to avoid the B virus, which is present in the hepatitis B vaccine, although in a weakened state. Also the B vaccine is full of a chemical called thimerosal which is full of mercury. Only two single-antigen pediatric hepatitis B vaccines exist on the US market, Engerix-B (SmithKline Beecham) and Recombivax HB (Merck). Both contain thimerosal and 12.5 micrograms of mercury per 0.5 ml dose.

Also avoid the flu shot, which stresses the immune system and raises viral load.

PRESCRIPTION DRUGS TO AVOID:

Certain prescription drugs should also be avoided.

AVOID NEXIUM, Prilosec and all acid pump inhibitors. These will raise your viral load millions of points overnight. No, it is not written in a medical journal that I know of but I have been observing this for many years.

AVOID AMOXICILLIN and all antibiotics. Amoxocillin will raise your viral load millions of points over night. Most antibiotics will cause problems in hepatitis C including but not limited to liver failure.

AVOID ANTIDEPRESSANTS. Over half of my clients are taking some kind of antidepressants. These drugs were originally designed to be taken for up to 3 months. After that, what people tell me is that they no longer cry but they also no longer laugh, do not enjoy sex, food, life etc. Many of them will raise your AST and ALT. Wellbutrin SR is the one I see raise liver enzymes the most. Zoloft, Paxil, Celexa, Effexor XR also raise the AST and ALT as well as the viral load.

AVOID VIAGRA. Studies show that the active ingredients in Viagra raise the viral load. For years I had clients who took Viagra and their viral loads rose slowly over time. There was nothing I could do to get them to go down. Then a client sent me a study showing clearly that Viagra raises the viral load in HCV. I sent a copy to the American Liver Foundation as they advocate the use of Viagra for liver transplant recipients. I have never heard back from them.

AVOID TYLENOL. Acetaminophen causes three times as many cases of liver failure as all other drugs combined. It is metabolized in the liver, resulting in a damaging chemical byproduct usually neutralized by glutathione. However, large doses of acetaminophen can overwhelm the body's natural supply of glutathione, resulting in the destruction of liver cells. Other medications containing acetaminophen include Excedrin, Midol, Alka-Seltzer, Theraflu, and Nyquil. Manufacturers of Tylenol recommend against taking two or more products containing acetaminophen at the same time.

FIBROSIS

Fibrosis is a scarring process that represents the liver's natural response to injury. Fibrosis itself is often classified stages 1 thru 4. Stage 4 is considered the beginning of cirrhosis. It can take years to move through these stages and you can live just fine in this condition if you eat right and take the right supplements.

CIRRHOSIS

Cirrhosis is a heavy scarring of the liver in which the architectural organization of the functional units of the liver become disrupted and blood flow through the liver and liver function become compromised. As the hepatitis C virus invades liver cells, your immune system tries to kill the virus and kills liver cells as a result. Over time this leads to cirrhosis. The average time to develop cirrhosis is about 30 years. Some people with hepatitis C never develop cirrhosis and others will develop cirrhosis faster than average.

Using milk thistle can strengthen liver cell walls and possibly delay this chronic condition.

A recent study shows that Mesenchyme may be able to stop or delay cirrhosis. BBC News reported on September 29, 2007, that scientists "have developed a new way to treat liver failure by dampening the immune response using a stem cell called Mesenchyme." At the time of the news release, the technique had only been used in animals. If it proves to be effective in humans, it could help save lives.

While the liver is one of the few major organs that is capable of regenerating itself, it cannot cope with the extensive damage it incurs from diseases such as chronic hepatitis or excessive long-term alcohol consumption. Natcell Mesenchyme can help diminish cell damage caused by the body's immune response.

PORTAL HYPERTENSION AND VARICES

As cirrhosis develops, the blood flow through the liver diminishes and pressure backs blood up into the esophagus and spleen. This pressure weakens and enlarges veins in the esophagus causing varices.

Esophageal varices are enlarged veins in the lower esophagus. They're often due to obstructed blood flow through the portal vein, an important blood vessel which carries blood from the intestine and spleen to the liver. This is a life-threatening condition. If these veins rupture, one can bleed to death rapidly.

An endoscopy is used to detect varices. If you have cirrhosis, get checked regularly. Banding is one procedure used to treat varices. Mesenchyme can also help this condition.

ASCITES

Ascites is a leakage of lymphatic fluid from the liver into the abdomen, and it is a devastating consequence of hepatitis C. The medical community prescribes diuretics, they mechanically remove lymphatic fluid from the abdomen with needles, but the only complete cure in serious cases is a liver transplant.

Over the past 12 years I have discovered that Natcell Thymus, Liver and Mesenchyme can be a successful treatment for Ascites. Three doses of Natcell Thymus, Liver and Mesenchyme a day can reverse Ascites.

LIVER CANCER

Liver cancer is one of the few cancers in the country that is on the rise, and this trend is expected to continue over the next two decades. Liver cancer or hepatocellular carcinoma affects over 750,000 people worldwide, with more than an estimated 20,000 new cases reported annually in the United States. For patients with cirrhosis, frequent surveillance is recommended, although current procedures are flawed.

Liver cancer in the US is almost always associated with chronic liver disease, according to the Liver Cancer Network. According to the American Association for the Study of Liver Diseases, hepatitis C infection is involved in more than half the cases of liver cancer. Survival is "significantly better for those who were asymptomatic at presentation or who were candidates for liver transplantation," said Dr. Alex S. Befeler of St. Louis University, Missouri. He added that chemotherapy is generally ineffective for liver cancer, since most patients are already suffering from advanced cirrhosis and therefore drug metabolism is poor. Transplantation offers the best approach, Dr. Befeler believes. [14]

In 2004, vitamin K made news as a possible preventive of liver cancer. A genetic link for the disease was identified in mice by researchers at the University of Illinois in Chicago. When the Foxm1b gene was deleted from liver cells in mice, the animals did not develop tumors, and they even remained cancer-free when the researchers used artificial means to induce tumors.

Research at the Houston VA Medical Center in Texas reported that diabetes increases the risk of serious liver problems, and that men with diabetes "have about a two-fold greater risk of developing liver cancer and other chronic liver diseases compared with non-diabetic men." [15]

Comitris, a liquid marine cartilage extract, is effective at treating primary liver cancer. Comitris can stop angiogenesis, the development of new blood vessels that feed tumors and allow them to grow and spread. Go to *www.comitris.net* and watch the learning module for more information.

NEW PEPTIDES MAY INHIBIT HEP C

One of the major stumbling blocks to developing a viable treatment for hepatitis C is the rapid rate at which the virus mutates and becomes drug resistant. But in the future, new compounds now undergoing study may be available.

The quest to find new treatments for the hepatitis C virus has led scientists from the Florida campus of The Scripps Research Institute and Boston University to discover "several novel drug-like inhibitors" with the "potential to substantially widen the current options to treat HCV infection," according to a December 21, 2009 report.

"With more than 170 million people infected worldwide by HCV, new therapeutic strategies are urgently needed for this blood-borne disease," researchers stated.

In seeking to reduce the rate of virus mutation, Dr. Strosberg of Scripps Florida and his colleagues have developed new compounds that not only "inhibited dimerization of the core, but also inhibited propagation of HCV in isolated hepatoma cells."

In an article the same year in the *Journal of General Virology*, Dr. Strosberg and a colleague described the process by which peptides derived from the HCV core protein also inhibited its dimerization.

A March 16, 2009 article in *Science Daily* reported that Dr. Strosberg and his team of researchers discovered two peptides that inhibited HCB production by 68% and 63%. A third related peptide showed 50% inhibition. "When added to HCV-infected cells, each of the three peptides blocked release but not replication of infectious virus; viral RNA levels were reduced by seven fold."

Confirmation of this study came from Frank Chisari of Scripps Research in La Jolla, California, who had been studying similar peptides, but using a different approach.

It is important to note that my Natcell formula is comprised of peptides. Check the product line at *www.AlternativeMedicineSolution.com* or call 1-877-676-1615 with any questions.

HEPATITIS C AND "BRAIN FOG"

In Canada, research scientists at the University of Alberta have recently discovered that the hepatitis C virus can breach the blood-brain barrier and lead to neuron damage as well as inflammation which stops the natural process of expelling toxins from brain cells called autophagy.

"For a long time, the medical community has recognized some people who have hepatitis C also have memory loss and poor concentration, which is very disabling for those patients," said Chris Power, who led the Canadian research team. "Now we have some understanding about the cause of these neurological symptoms that can lead to the development of future treatments for people with hepatitis C." [16]

This Canadian study suggests that 13 percent of the 300,000 Canadians with hepatitis C also have neurological problems. The hepatitis C virus damages those neurons in the brain responsible for motor functions, memory and concentration. There is nonetheless hope, since growth factors linked to the regeneration mechanism of nerves are rapidly being identified.

Natcell CNS is the only item I have seen that has been effective at reducing these kinds of serious problems. The central nervous system and lungs of porcine embryos are naturally rich sources of neurotrophic factors.

Because of the discovery of neurotrophic factors, it is now possible to hope that nerve cell lesions caused by the hepatitis C virus are reversible. Growth factors make it possible to improve the regeneration of injured nerves and neurons of the nervous system. The therapeutic effects of neurotrophic factors are extremely promising.

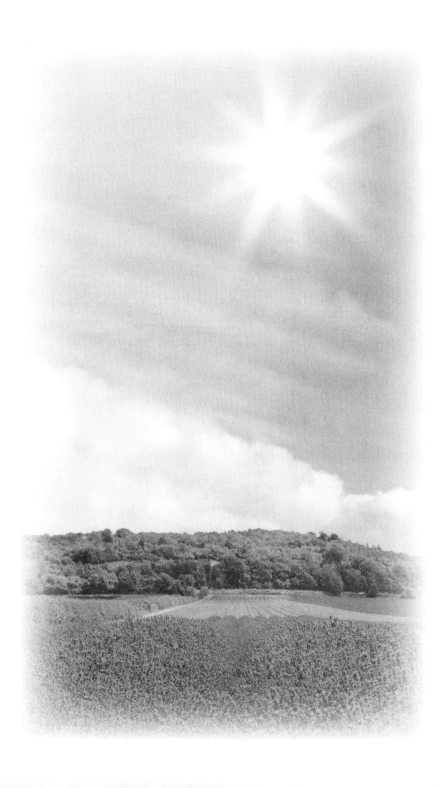

Chapter 5

FREQUENTLY ASKED QUESTIONS

Q — *Why does my viral load go up and down?*

A — Most often a secondary condition is the cause. A simple bacterial infection, mild virus, or a sore throat can cause havoc. These *secondary conditions* can make one feel sick and fatigued on a range from mild to severe. This can be short lived or last for months. The biggest and most dangerous problem that now enters is the Mad Doctor.

Many of these people prescribe antibiotics, which will make the problem much worse, and often they do not check to see if a bacteria is responsible and often it is not. In these situations, avoid antibiotics and use Ultra-Absorbic vitamin

C, colloidal silver, and Natcell Thymus. At the onset of a cold or flu infection, take **Oregacillin** 450 mg. and/or **Lysine** 3000 mg.

Vaccines such as those for hepatitis A and B, flu shots, and tetanus will all raise your viral load dramatically – please see Chapter 4.

Nexium, the prescription purple pill, Prilosec, and other acid pump inhibitors, will cause a dramatic rise in your viral load. Use Zantac or Tums, instead.

Some people have a viral load that fluctuates. After Peg-Intron or Roche's Pegasus, the viral load will escalate to three times baseline and more. Most will see a peak about two years after the last shot.

Plane travel can raise your viral load. The cabin pressure is always lower than what atmospheric pressure would be on the ground on long flights. When exposed to this condition for long periods of time, the result is a surge in viral load.

Learn where your viral load lives and get acquainted with it. Don't fear it. Conquer it. Do not obsess over it...PRAY!

Q — *Why is my ALT and AST high?*

A — About two-thirds of my clients have elevated ALT and AST. Many have normal liver enzymes for decades, then they encounter an MD who prescribes antidepressants, antibiotics, and vaccines. The ones I see have elevated ALT and AST and most are on Wellbutrin SR, Lexapro, Effexor XR, Serzone, Celexa, and Zoloft, with Wellbutrin SR being the worst. Also, antibiotics will raise the AST and ALT. Antibiotics are found in pills, capsules, eye drops, suppositories, and Perio Chips. Pain pills, sedatives, tranquilizers, and sleeping pills will also compromise ALT and AST.

Once the basic reference range is compromised from using many of these drugs, the ALT and AST range jumps to between 80 and 120 as an average for most with hepatitis C. A smaller percentage will round off between 180 and 280.

In the early stages of hepatitis C, it is fairly easy to lower your numbers. In the later stages, it is far more difficult.

What you need to know is that, for most people, a range of 80-120 is not a death sentence, and you can live with it. Work on lowering these numbers, but do not become obsessed with them. Worry kills!

Always use the five items in my Program One

as a minimum. To increase your chances, take two or three Liver Formula II before breakfast with two Blueberry Extract 45% proanthocyanidin with one 5 mg. NADH. Take two or three Apolactoferrin (iron removed) with one Phosphatidyl Choline before bed.

Sweating and exercising keep your lymph system moving and remove many of the toxins developed by hepatitis. **Body movement is the driver that propels your lymph system.**

Remember, the hepatitis C virus itself damages liver cells and will raise your AST and ALT.

Q — *What is Ferritin?*

A — Ferritin is a form of iron stored mostly in the liver. About a third of people with hepatitis C will have high ferritin. Most MDs will not routinely test for this. However, high ferritin can be responsible for some of your symptoms. Most of the time removing high ferritin will remove these symptoms, and your life should return to normal.

The hardest part of dealing with high ferritin is finding a doctor who will recognize it as a problem, a treatable one. Go to an understanding hematologist (blood doctor).

For most of us, reducing ferritin levels to normal requires regular therapeutic phlebotomies. When we stop, ferritin goes up and it requires a lot of work to lower it back.

In order to be a candidate for therapeutic phlebotomy, your platelets must be normal. If platelets are low, use Norwegian shark liver oil 1000 mg. per day for thirty days, which should raise your platelets 20-26 points.

There are some standard written theories on ferritin removal that lead doctors to bunch therapeutic phlebotomies close together and lead you into anemia. WRONG for us!

If you cannot have a therapeutic phlebotomy, as an alternative use Inositol Hexaphosphate or IP-6. Understand that IP-6 is slow and success varies.

Q — *Does Ozone therapy work?*

A — Ozone therapy is done in several different ways. Routinely I see better success from ozone therapy done in Mexico than what is done in the US. This is in part due to laws regarding the procedure in the US restricting how it is done.

When done properly ozone can lower the AST and ALT. When one stops generally the AST and ALT revert to baseline.

Q — What do I do for bladder infections?

A — Over 90% of all urinary tract infections are caused by *Escherichia coli (E. coli)* bacteria which are part of the normal microflora in every intestinal tract. In most cases bacteria enter the urinary tract through the urethral opening. Most bacteria are simply washed away by the down-flow of urine. E. coli, however, are covered with tiny 'finger-like' projections. At the top of these projections are amino acid/sugar complexes called "lectins" which allow the bacteria to stick to the inside walls of the urinary tract and even work their way upward.

The answer to this is D-Mannose, a naturally occurring simple sugar which sticks to the E. coli lectins even better than the lectins stick to human cells. When a large quantity of this sugar is present in the urine, it literally coats any E. coli present. They can no longer stick to urinary tract walls and are washed away with normal urination. Only very small amounts of D-mannose are metabolized by the body. Most is excreted through the kidneys into the urine and bladder, so it doesn't interfere with blood sugar regulation, even in people with diabetes. Also, since it is absorbed in the upper gastro-intestinal tract, it does not relocate "friendly"

E. coli or other beneficial bacteria normally present in the colon.

Please try D-Mannose before resorting to antibiotics. It works nearly every time.

Q — Should I get the flu shot?

A — NO! First, the evidence shows that flu shots do not work. When one has hepatitis C, taking the flu shot puts a load on your immune system, raises your viral load and compromises your immune system.

Q — *Why do I get cramps?*

A — In hepatitis, cramps, especially in the legs, can be severe and very painful. Take some potassium citrate 100 mg. 3x day until symptoms stop.

Q — *What is fever therapy?*

A — When a virus is subjected to temperatures of 102 degrees inside the body, the virus begins to die off. There are various ways to achieve this condition. A hot tub with a water temperature of 106 degrees for 30 minutes can raise your internal body temperature to 102 degrees. Then you follow this with 30 minutes in an infrared sauna with internal temperature of 106 degrees.

I have several clients that pay enormous amounts of money for this therapy. They tell me that while they use this therapy their viral load drops tens of thousands of points. However, the virus does inch up when they stop.

You can purchase a good infrared sauna and a hot tub and do this at home. Be sure you do not do this alone and drink plenty of water. Additional things to incorporate are taking Natcell Thymus prior to doing this, also ultra Absorbic Vitamin C may help destroy hepatitis C virus.

Chapter 6

LETTERS

Every day I hear stories from victims of hepatitis C that would be dismissed as fiction by the medical community, not to mention the average American. A good number of their stories are even more dramatic than my own personal account.

In this book, I have included only a small sampling of the feedback I have received from my readers. I hope that these testimonials will inspire hope in hepatitis C sufferers and instill in them the determination necessary for their ultimate survival.

I recently heard from a 42-year-old client in Arizona who underwent gallbladder surgery. During the procedure, she had a liver biopsy, which revealed hepatitis C, stage 2 cirrhosis. Her hepatologist told her that her condition was too severe to treat with interferon, and that she would need a liver transplant.

After some research, the woman read the first edition of *Triumph Over Hepatitis C*. She liked what she saw, and tried the program. After three months, she returned to her doctor at the University of Arizona Teaching Hospital. He was surprised to see her looking so healthy.

When he learned she was taking herbs, he immediately became defensive and said he must have made a mistake with her earlier diagnosis. He said, "You cannot get well from this condition."

A 40-year-old woman called me and sounded as though she were near death. She told me that following my program had cured her friend, and that she needed my help because her medical doctor was "killing" her with four years of interferon treatment. After revealing to me the number of tests she had been taking, I concluded she was being used as a guinea pig in order to determine the long-term effects of interferon. She was a perfect victim, in that she did not suffer the usual hard effects associated with interferon. When she pleaded with the doctor to stop the treatment, he warned her she would die without it.

After speaking with me, she stopped the treatment on her own, and went on my program. The positive effects began immediately.

Below are sections of an email exchange that is currently going on with one of my Ascites clients. This shows day-to-day how well taking Natcell for this condition works. This is a very famous man who was extremely skeptical. His wife got the Natcell for him as a last resort and kept me updated about his progress.

Day 1

Thanks so much! I so appreciate your guidance through this process. FYI, so far, so good. Today was day 1 and he's not even itching (he was itching like crazy all week last week, I think due to the sulfa in the endocrin, but also as to the total imbalance of the liver itself). He's really amazed, as am I!

Day 4

Well here we are at the end of day 4 and his edema is slowly but surely dissipating thank goodness. His itching is gone, he's losing 3-4 lbs. a day and is feeling better overall. Can't wait to see what happens at day 24!!! I know, it's making me so crazy, I want to scream and cry from frustration, more out of the fact that he doesn't seem to want to believe, even though it's happening in front of his very eyes!!! Last night he claimed it's the diuretics pulling the weight off him—I let him in on my little secret that I cut his dosage of that stuff to 1/4 of what he was told to take so he could have semi-regular bowel movements. He was angry with me and incredulous that I would have the audacity to defy the doctors like that and take his life into my hands. The other night he looked at me in total skepticism on the entire process he's doing and said "Are you willing to risk my life with this stuff?" and I responded, after about a half a beat, "Yes." He just shook his head at me.

Day 8

His itching is occasionally returning at night, and his edema comes and goes (never to the extent it was though—elephantitis), but overall he says he's feeling better. I keep having to remind him that this stuff IS working. He's completed 8 days on this protocol and he seems to think that he should be much better by now. I keep having to remind him that Rome was not built in a day, and true it took but a few days to tear it down, it takes much more time to rebuild, patience, patience, patience (which he has none). You get the idea.

I think given the fact that he's only been on it for 8 days and has lost 14 pounds is significant. Also he's feeling more lucid, less angry and hostile, more functional and inclined to be active. All good signs I think. He's not working out again like he should be but he will at some point.

Day 15

Yesterday he was itching terribly (I think it's the Edecrin-diuretic, talked him into not taking it for a day or two just to see if maybe the itching would subside—he's got an allergy to sulfa drugs, duh), weight was 212, up from 210 (I take increases in weight to mean we're going backwards not for-wards) and I was beginning to feel hopeless as we near day 15 on this protocol. This morning, blood pressure still perfect, his weight is down to 205!!! Same scale! Woohoo!

Ascites is diminishing to be sure (he now has flaps of skin where before it was completely taut), so I know that's going away. He still does have edema, although not nearly as bad. You're quite right, it probably did take years to acquire—and I do believe some of it was alcohol related. His favorite drink not long ago and for as long as I've known him was Wild Turkey (19 years at the least).

Day 24

He is doing so great, really! So much so (as I'd hoped), he's ordered another set. And I anticipate that by the time he's starting this new series, he's going to feel better than he has in years. So so so grateful to you, Lloyd. Wish I could hug you! Sending you an internet one anyway!

Hi, Lloyd,

Just wanted to share the news. I have cleared the virus. Thanks for all your kindness and support.

— Lisa R.

Lloyd,

So after everything that went on here is the latest:

Brother John went into his GI doctor and they could not believe their eyes. As it was only 2 months ago that they told him he had Ascites and a failing liver and he could get his affairs in order. I kept telling him to order the Nat Cell and take it every day if he could afford it, he did and continues. They did a scan and blood work and all tests are in the normal

*range now, yes incredible. This is the huge one.........
his Ascites is gone too, yes I know Ascites does not
go away but his did. He only takes 1 or so water
pills each week instead of 5 per day. He has gained
NO water weight and stomach is flat. More over his
GI doctor said he does not know what he is doing
but keep it up. The GI said NO on liver issues. The
doctor who does renal medicine said kidneys are
good. They did a test yesterday by putting a camera
down his throat and found no varices at all or any
large veins. They also said everything looks excellent
down there. I am also going to tell you Thank you
for helping John, he is very grateful for you having
the Nat Cell and very appreciative of you being so
honest and forthright in helping him. I also am always grateful to you as you have done so much for
our family. I know your techniques saved his life.*

—David, Washington

John had serious Ascites. He was told his time
had come. He took Natcell Thymus, Natcell Liver
and Natcell Mesenchyme every day for two months
and above are the results.

I have had similar results with hundreds of terminal cases.

—Lloyd

Hi, Lloyd!

I really can't express how much your program means to me—I mean it's my LIFE! I am a 39 year-old female. I found out I had this [HCV] last summer and was obsessed with the seemingly endless ramifications—it felt like my life was truly over. I took some of the supplements, but started on almost all of the program in February (all except cat's claw and hyssop teas and I dropped Hepastat in March, so really all of it.) Like most, I had horrible experiences with a gastroenterologist who really pushed for a biopsy and touted the benefits of pegylated interferon, which would "knock the virus out of me." I knew, from you, that the only thing that would be knocked out was me, so I went for the ultrasound which said no damage was found and refused the biopsy—there was no reason for it, and that would definitely cause scarring to the liver. Your site has given me endless hope, especially lately as more great test results come in… Anyway, to everyone out there—keep plugging—IT WORKS! If insurance would pay for this program, think of how much it would save them in the long run. I'm, faxing the labs to you, and am just THRILLED about the results! Thanks again.

— S

Debra Caprianos wrote me a very moving letter about her husband's struggle with hepatitis C, which makes the vital point that time is of the essence. After her husband passed away, Debra wrote, *"During the last week of his life my frantic research led me to four different methods of helping his condition, one of which was yours... But unfortunately it was...too late... Thanks for being the champion you are!"*

I have received countless letters over the years from satisfied clients, along with the positive results from their lab tests following the use of the program outlined in this book. These letters remain in my files as a living testament to the fact that the supplements in this book can pave the way to optimal health.

Don't waste time worrying about money. Spend your time making more time. Take action now!

Chapter 7

CLOSING
THOUGHTS

Hepatitis C is a life-threatening virus, but doctors are still treating their patients with interferon, even though this "therapy" and all its combinations have proven to be a complete failure. With all the research studies performed over these past two decades, medical science is still without a viable treatment.

Rather than recognize the value of natural therapies, medical doctors recommend little else to their patients other than to wait for a liver transplant. Many die waiting. Still more die from the complications of hepatitis C which cannot be helped by a donor liver.

Fortunately, in the 21st century, man has rediscovered time-proven options in natural healing. As a culture, we are becoming more aware of the fact that we can support our immune system and help it achieve what it was designed specifically to do—heal our bodies.

I believe that with knowledge and persistence we can achieve optimum health. Unfortunately, it takes time, money, and sacrifice to learn about and acquire the necessary natural herbal supplements.

Over the past forty years, the prevailing health care system and the government agencies entrusted to regulate it have virtually excluded treatments related to so-called alternative, traditional, or unorthodox medicine. Especially kept in competitive check have been herbs and other nutritional supplements, which hundreds of studies have demonstrated possess the potential to replace many modern synthesized pharmaceutical drugs. The repression of health care alternatives has been achieved both directly through regulatory control and indirectly through what would appear to be a systematic offensive against alternative health care providers.

The government has required that any time there is a health claim about an herb or dietary supplement, the producer must prove that the supplement is safe and effective. While this seems fair enough, the reality is that a new drug application costs up to $359 million and takes eight years or more to process. Pharmaceutical companies are rewarded for their investments by receiving patents on their drugs. Most ironically, a whole herb is a natural substance that cannot be patented. It is somewhat of a foreign concept in this era of modern medicine's magic bullets to imagine that nutrition, herbs, and supplements benefit so many parts of the body.

Alternative medicine means that there is another option in medicinal treatment, particularly when the ones we are accustomed to relying on prove ineffective. While I may seem at times in opposition to modern medicine, the fact is that my skepticism has been forced upon me simply by my choice to be open to the credible healing benefits of herbs and nutritional supplements. Actually, I hope that both conventional and alternative medicine can unite and thus expand, enabling people to choose their path of treatment while being supported by their insurance companies and physicians.

In the case of hepatitis C, it is a proven fact that what the medical community is offering as treatment at this time still does not work, and, in fact, exacerbates the condition. When I was diagnosed with hepatitis C, I turned first to conventional medicine for healing. When the prescribed treatment of interferon not only did not work, but actually made me sicker, I had no choice but to explore and self-prescribe a treatment of natural remedies that ultimately became my cure.

AVOID MEDICAL DOCTORS

My experience taught me that those people who attach "M.D." to their names should be avoided completely during the healing process from hepatitis C. After reading this book, in which I attempted to summarize my thoughts, you will likely understand why I feel as I do.

Medical doctors are very expensive and know nothing about nutritional support or natural healing. However, if you reach the stage of requiring a liver transplant, the medical doctor is your only recourse. Choose wisely—select one who is a good mechanic and who has a good access to a supply of available livers.

In closing my argument against medical doctors, I offer these staggering figures: a recent study by the Hearst Corporation estimated that almost 200,000 Americans die annually from preventable medical mistakes, making this the third leading cause of death in the U.S.—ahead of traffic accidents, breast cancer, and AIDS. This figure is almost four times higher than the number of American soldiers killed during all the years of the Vietnam War. Dr. Sid Wolfe of Public Citizen, a consumer watchdog group, has asserted that medical errors have been buried too long, and it's time they were all reported to public agencies.

Pharmaceutical companies also have a way of coming up with a new drug to "cure" hepatitis C every 6-12 months. This causes nothing but confusion in the hepatitis C community. The "cure" hoopla starts with news reports or press releases claiming spectacular results in trials conducted in third world countries, reports which always include the company's stock symbol and related financial information. The HCV "cure" is hyped in the press for months, people are informed of coming trials and possible FDA approvals, stock prices surge 600%, but after a while talk of the alleged "cure" just disappears. I never bother to keep track of this hype, but one example comes to mind. Around the turn of the century, Amgen claimed to have a "cure" for hepatitis C which got a lot of press and didn't pan out. And at this writing, Vertex Pharmaceuticals and Merck are moving ahead with the new drugs telaprevir and boceprevir which are to be combined with pharmaceutical interferon and ribavirin for the first three months of treatment. This is likely to be much to do about nothing.

SHARING MY THERAPY

Personally, having shared my therapy with thousands of hepatitis C victims, I know with certainty that what worked for me also works for others. It is therefore my opinion, based on the results reported to me, that this program works better than anything currently offered by the FDA.

To view hundreds of testimonials, read my book *Hepatitis C Free, Alternative Medicine vs. The Drug Industry, The People Speak*. If you have any doubt about anything written in the book you are now reading, that book provides numerous testimonials that should answer any of your concerns.

A good solid belief in God, a structured lifestyle, and heightened self-awareness are necessary prerequisites for success in all aspects of life. If you are not satisfied with your current level of discipline in the area of health, now is the time to get motivated to save your life.

Appendix A:

MEDICAL TESTS

The following medical tests are often given to people with hepatitis C. Results of some tests may vary considerably, but can be helpful in monitoring your progress over time.

HEPATITIS C GENOTYPES

Isolates of hepatitis C virus are now grouped into six major genotypes. These are sub-typed according to sequence characteristics and are designated as 1a, 1b, 1c, 2a, 2b, 2c, 3a, 3b, 4a-h, and 6a. Medical doctors believe certain genotypes have better results with interferon treatment than others. For example, genotypes 2 and 3 are now believed two or three times more likely to respond to interferon treatment than genotype 1. Interferon is typically given by doctors for 24 weeks to genotypes 2 and 3, and for 48 weeks to genotype 1.

LIVER FUNCTION TESTS:

AST (SGOT)

The AST is a liver function test that measures liver enzymes and inflammation.

In blood tests, increases in aspartate aminotransferase or AST, a protein normally found inside liver cells, are seen in any condition involving necrosis or death of hepatocytes, myocardial cells, or skeletal muscle cells.

ALT (SGPT)

The ALT is another liver function test that measures liver enzymes and inflammation.

Increased serum alanine aminotransferase or ALT, another protein normally found inside liver cells, is seen in any condition involving necrosis or death of hepatocytes, myocardial cells, erythrocytes, or skeletal muscle cells.

BILIRUBIN

Serum total bilirubin is increased in liver cell or hepatocellular damage (infectious hepatitis, alcoholic, and other toxic hepatopathy, neoplasmas), and intra- and extra-hepatic biliary tract obstruction.

ALBUMIN

Albumin is an important protein made in the liver. Decreased amounts of serum albumin or albumin in the blood are seen when the liver does not manufacture sufficient amounts or too much albumin is excreted from the body leading to malnutrition or mal-absorption of nutrients in conjunction with liver disease or other chronic diseases.

PCR – POLYMERASE CHAIN REACTION (VIRAL LOAD)

This test is used to measure the viral load of the hepatitis C virus in the RNA. Hepatitis C is an RNA virus unlike most other viruses, which are DNA viruses.

Currently performed in many different ways, this test's results are often confusing and frustrating. Most doctors tell patients, "If it's over 850,000, it's bad." This is not true. The viral load of a specific person is not related to ALT and AST levels, symptoms, or liver damage.

When requesting a PCR, ask for "PCR HCV RNA QUANTITATIVE (VIRAL LOAD) — specific number". (New tests are constantly emerging. See message board for updates at the website *www.lloydwright.org*)

IRON PANEL

This is a very important test, often overlooked by doctors. You will not improve until your iron levels are in the normal range. High iron and or ferritin occurs in about 30% of men, 8% of pre-menopausal females and about 25% of post menopausal females who have hepatitis C. A therapeutic phlebotomy or drawing of blood is the best method to lower iron levels. Inositol hexaphosphate or IP-6 can work although it takes much longer. Within one to three months of normalizing your ferritin (see below) your ALT and AST should follow.

FERRITIN TEST

Ferritin is a complex of iron and protein mainly found in the liver. A ferritin test is more specific to the liver than an iron test for people with hepatitis C, since ferritin is the way the liver stores most of its iron. Please try to get both tests; tests should both be normal in order for your health to improve.

ALPHA FETA PROTEIN (AFP)

This protein is produced by people with hepatic carcinoma or germ cell tumors. Approximately 79-90% of people with hepatocellular carcinoma will have levels that range from above normal 20 ng/ml to 10,000,000 ng/ml. A small elevation in AFP may occur in people with non-malignant disease such as cirrhosis or viral hepatitis. This test should be accompanied with an ultrasound to confirm results. I recommend having this test and an ultrasound of the liver and gallbladder once a year.

PLATELET COUNT

Platelets help your blood clot and this test counts the number of platelets in your blood. If your platelet count drops below 140, use Norwegian Shark Liver Oil to raise it.

FIBROSURE BLOOD TEST

HCV Fibrosure is a noninvasive blood test that combines the quantitative results of six serum biochemical markers. Using a patented algorithm analyzing six serum biochemical markers, HCV Fibrosure has been shown to lead to a reliable quantitative assessment of fibrogenic and inflammatory activity in the liver of HCV patients. It provides an accurate measure of bridging fibrosis and/or moderate necroinflammatory activity.

FOOTNOTES

1. Saito, H., et al., "Enhancing effect of the liver extract and flavin adenine Dinucleotide mixture on anti-viral efficacy of interferon in patients with chronic hepatitis C," *Keio Journal of Medicine*, Vol. 45, No. 1, pp. 48-53, March 1996.

2. Nelson, C., et al., "Giycerophosphoryiethanolamine (GPEA) identified as an hepatocyte growth stimulator in liver extracts," *Experimental Cell Research*, Vol. 229, No. 1, pp. 20-26, Nov. 1996.

3. Rohrer, Jean, "Healing Light: Milk Thistle," Internet *http://home.earthlink.net/~anitaastrologer/beathepc.htm*

4. Law, David, "Medical Mushrooms: An Ancient Alternative to Synthetic Drugs, A Positive Approach to Health and Wellness," *http://www.gmushrooms.com/health.htm*

5. Mowrey, Dan, "Licorice for the Female Reproductive System," *Health Store News*, June/July 1995.

6. Finnegan, Dr. John, *The Healing Aloe: Nature's Wondrous Gift and Cancer Prevention and Recover: A Nutritional Approach.*

7. Larsen, Hans R., "Vitamin C: Your Ultimate Health Insurance, *International Health News*. *http://www.yourhealthbase.com*

8. Grieve, Maud, *A Modern Herbal (Volume 1, A-H): The Medicinal, Culinary, Cosmetic and Economic Properties, Cultivation and Folk-Lore of Herbs, Grasses, Fungi, Shrubs & Trees with Their Modern Scientific Uses* (Jun 1, 1971)

9. Williams, S.R. *Nutrition and Diet Therapy*, C.W. Mosby Co., 1969.

10. Grieve, Maud, *A Modern Herbal (Volume 1, A-H): The Medicinal, Culinary, Cosmetic and Economic Properties, Cultivation and Folk-Lore of Herbs, Grasses, Fungi, Shrubs & Trees with Their Modern Scientific Uses*, pp. 105, 121, 129.

11. Shahani and Fernandes, "Anticarcinogenic and immune-logical properties of dietary lactobacilli," *Journal of Food Protection*, Vol. 53, pp. 704-711, 1990.

12. Oster, Kurt, "Milk: The Homogenization Deception," Internet 1999.

13. David Wraith, professor at University of Bristol, and Richard Daniels, Apitope company.

14. *Reuters Health*, January 11, 2004.

15. *Reuters Health*, February 25, 2004.

16. "U of A medical research team discovers hepatitis C virus damages brain cells, "University of Alberta Express News, *Public Library of Science One Journal*, Oct. 7, 2010.

LLOYD WRIGHT PUBLISHING

www.AlternativeMedicineSolution.com